Glycemic Index & Glycemic Load of Foods

2nd Edition

DietGrail.com

ISBN-13: 978-1463799717

Table of Contents

Introduction

This publication contains the glycemic index and glycemic load data for approximately 3,800 food items. The glycemic load is calculated based on 100g of food weight.

All information in this publication is available for free at DietGrail.com. In particular, our glycemic index webpage is useful if you need to search for specific foods or sort foods based on their glycemic index or glycemic load values or view other nutrient data.

Format of each entry: Glycemic Index, Glycemic Load followed by Food Name.
Abbreviation used:
NS = not specified

DietGrail Publisher
http://dietgrail.com

MILK and MILK PRODUCTS

Milk and Milk Drinks

GI	GL	Food Name
30	1.4	Milk
27	1.2	Milk, cow's, fluid, whole
31	1.4	Milk, cow's, fluid, whole, low-sodium
31	1.4	Milk, calcium fortified, cow's, fluid, whole
32	1.6	Milk, calcium fortified, cow's, fluid, 1% fat
32	1.6	Milk, calcium fortified, cow's, fluid, skim or nonfat
32	1.5	Milk, cow's, fluid, other than whole ("lowfat")
30	1.4	Milk, cow's, fluid, 2% fat
32	1.6	Milk, cow's, fluid, acidophilus, 1% fat
30	1.4	Milk, cow's, fluid, acidophilus, 2% fat
32	1.6	Milk, cow's, fluid, 1% fat
32	1.6	Milk, cow's, fluid, skim or nonfat, 0.5% or less butterfat
32	1.6	Milk, cow's, fluid, lactose reduced, 1% fat
32	1.6	Milk, cow's, fluid, lactose reduced, 1% fat, fortified with calcium
32	1.6	Milk, cow's, fluid, lactose reduced, nonfat
32	1.6	Milk, cow's, fluid, lactose reduced, nonfat, fortified with calcium
30	1.4	Milk, cow's, fluid, lactose reduced, 2% fat
31	1.4	Milk, cow's, fluid, lactose reduced, whole
32	1.5	Buttermilk, fluid, nonfat
31	1.5	Buttermilk, fluid, 1% fat
30	1.6	Buttermilk, fluid, 2% fat

MILK and MILK PRODUCTS

GI	GL	Food Name
27	1.2	Milk, goat's, fluid, whole
32	1.6	Milk, dry, reconstituted
27	1.3	Milk, dry, reconstituted, whole
32	1.6	Milk, dry, reconstituted, lowfat
32	1.6	Milk, dry, reconstituted, nonfat
27	1.4	Milk, evaporated
27	2.7	Milk, evaporated, used in coffee or tea (assume
27	2.7	Milk, evaporated, undiluted
27	1.4	Milk, evaporated, diluted
27	1.4	Milk, evaporated, whole
27	2.7	Milk, evaporated, whole, used in coffee or tea
27	2.7	Milk, evaporated, whole, undiluted
27	1.4	Milk, evaporated, whole, diluted
27	3.0	Milk, evaporated, 2% fat
27	3.0	Milk, evaporated, 2% fat, undiluted
27	1.6	Milk, evaporated, 2% fat, diluted
32	1.9	Milk, evaporated, skim
32	3.6	Milk, evaporated, skim, used in coffee or tea
32	3.6	Milk, evaporated, skim, undiluted
32	1.9	Milk, evaporated, skim, diluted
61	33.2	Milk, condensed, sweetened
61	33.2	Milk, condensed, sweetened, undiluted
61	18.7	Milk, condensed, sweetened, diluted
40	1.5	Milk, soy, ready-to-drink, not baby's

GI	GL	Food Name
40	2.3	Milk, soy, ready-to-drink, not baby's, chocolate
33	6.2	Yogurt
32	2.2	Yogurt, plain
36	1.7	Yogurt, plain, whole milk
36	2.5	Yogurt, plain, lowfat milk
36	2.8	Yogurt, plain, nonfat milk
27	3.7	Yogurt, vanilla, lemon, or coffee flavor
27	3.7	Yogurt, vanilla, lemon, or coffee flavor, whole milk
27	3.7	Yogurt, vanilla, lemon, maple, or coffee flavor, lowfat
32	5.6	Yogurt, vanilla, lemon, maple, or coffee flavor, nonfat
19	1.4	Yogurt, vanilla, lemon, maple, or coffee flavor, nonfat milk, sweetened with low calorie sweetener
33	7.8	Yogurt, chocolate
32	7.3	Yogurt, chocolate, whole milk
32	7.5	Yogurt, chocolate, nonfat milk
33	6.3	Yogurt, fruit variety
33	6.1	Yogurt, fruit variety, whole milk
31	5.9	Yogurt, fruit variety, lowfat milk
25	4.7	Yogurt, fruit variety, lowfat milk, sweetened with low-calorie sweetener
32	6.1	Yogurt, fruit variety, nonfat milk
19	1.5	Yogurt, fruit variety, nonfat milk, sweetened with low-calorie sweetener
50	9.8	Yogurt, frozen
50	9.6	Yogurt, frozen, flavors other than chocolate

MILK and MILK PRODUCTS

GI	GL	Food Name
50	10.8	Yogurt, frozen, chocolate
50	9.8	Yogurt, frozen, lowfat milk
50	10.8	Yogurt, frozen, chocolate, lowfat milk
50	9.6	Yogurt, frozen, flavors other than chocolate, lowfat milk
50	11.0	Yogurt, frozen, nonfat milk
50	11.1	Yogurt, frozen, chocolate, nonfat milk
50	12.6	Yogurt, frozen, flavors other than chocolate, with sorbet or sorbet-coated
50	9.8	Yogurt, frozen, flavors other than chocolate, nonfat milk
50	9.9	Yogurt, frozen, chocolate, nonfat milk, with low-calorie sweetener
50	14.1	Yogurt, frozen, flavors other than chocolate, nonfat milk, with low-calorie sweetener
50	10.8	Yogurt, frozen, whole milk
50	10.8	Yogurt, frozen, chocolate, whole milk
50	10.8	Yogurt, frozen, flavors other than chocolate, whole milk
50	14.5	Yogurt, frozen, chocolate-coated
50	15.7	Yogurt, frozen, carob-coated
50	18.8	Yogurt, frozen, sandwich
50	15.7	Yogurt, frozen, cone, chocolate
50	15.8	Yogurt, frozen, cone, flavors other than chocolate
50	5.6	Yogurt, frozen, cone, flavors other than chocolate, lowfat milk
50	12.5	Yogurt, frozen, cone, chocolate, lowfat milk
37	4.3	Milk, chocolate

GI	GL	Food Name
36	3.7	Milk, chocolate, whole milk-based
38	4.5	Milk, chocolate, reduced fat milk-based, 2% ("lowfat")
38	4.1	Milk, chocolate, skim milk-based
37	3.9	Milk, chocolate, lowfat milk-based
36	4.3	Cocoa, hot chocolate, not from dry mix, made with whole milk
37	4.4	Cocoa and sugar mixture, milk added
36	4.2	Cocoa and sugar mixture, whole milk added
37	4.4	Cocoa and sugar mixture, reduced fat milk added
38	4.5	Cocoa and sugar mixture, lowfat milk added
38	4.5	Cocoa and sugar mixture, skim milk added
36	4.6	Chocolate syrup, milk added
36	4.5	Chocolate syrup, whole milk added
36	4.6	Chocolate syrup, reduced fat milk added
36	4.7	Chocolate syrup, lowfat milk added
38	4.9	Chocolate syrup, skim milk added
38	4.3	Cocoa, sugar, and dry milk mixture, water added
24	1.3	Cocoa with nonfat dry milk and low calorie sweetener, mixture, water added
24	1.6	Cocoa, whey, and low-calorie sweetener mixture, lowfat milk added
24	1.3	Milk beverage with nonfat dry milk and low calorie sweetener, water added, chocolate
24	1.5	Milk beverage with nonfat dry milk and low calorie sweetener, water added, flavors other than chocolate

MILK and MILK PRODUCTS

GI	GL	Food Name
24	1.3	Milk beverage with nonfat dry milk and low calorie sweetener, high calcium, water added, chocolate
35	4.3	Milk beverage, made with whole milk, flavors other than chocolate
35	4.3	Milk, flavors other than chocolate, whole milk-based
45	5.0	Milk, malted, unfortified, made with milk
45	5.0	Milk, malted, unfortified, chocolate, made with milk
45	5.2	Milk, malted, unfortified, chocolate, made with skim milk
45	4.5	Milk, malted, unfortified, natural flavor, made with milk
45	5.0	Milk, malted, fortified, natural flavor, made with milk
45	5.0	Milk, malted, fortified, chocolate, made with milk
45	5.0	Milk, malted, fortified, made with milk
44	8.8	Milk shake
44	8.9	Milk shake, homemade or fountain-type
44	9.4	Milk shake, homemade or fountain-type, chocolate
44	9.4	Milk shake, homemade or fountain-type, flavors other than chocolate
53	11.4	Milk shake with malt
47	10.4	Milk shake, made with skim milk, chocolate
47	10.1	Milk shake, made with skim milk, flavors other than chocolate
44	8.8	Carry-out milk shake
44	9.0	Carry-out milk shake, chocolate
44	8.6	Carry-out milk shake, flavors other than chocolate
43	6.3	Orange Julius

GI	GL	Food Name
38	4.0	Chocolate-flavored drink, whey- and milk-based
35	3.7	Flavored milk drink, whey- and milk-based, flavors other than chocolate
26	3.3	Instant breakfast, fluid, canned
26	3.3	Instant breakfast, powder, milk added
26	1.9	Instant breakfast, powder, sweetened with low calorie sweetener, milk added
26	2.8	Diet beverage, liquid, canned
50	5.5	Meal supplement or replacement, commercially prepared, ready-to-drink
33	4.3	Meal supplement or replacement, milk-based, high protein, liquid
49	26.7	Meal replacement, high protein, milk based, fruit juice mixable formula, powdered, not reconstituted
49	31.1	Meal replacement, protein type, milk-based, powdered, not reconstituted
49	32.5	Nutrient supplement, milk-based, powdered, not reconstituted
49	9.1	Nutrient supplement, milk-based, high protein, powdered, not reconstituted

Cream and Cream Substitutes

GI	GL	Food Name
27	1.2	Cream, NS as to light, heavy, or half and half
27	1.0	Cream, light, fluid
27	0.8	Cream, light, whipped, unsweetened
27	1.2	Cream, half and half
27	2.4	Cream, half and half, fat free

MILK and MILK PRODUCTS

GI	GL	Food Name
27	0.8	Cream, heavy, fluid
55	4.7	Cream, heavy, whipped, sweetened
55	6.9	Cream, whipped, pressurized container
27	3.1	Cream substitute
27	3.1	Cream substitute, frozen
27	3.1	Cream substitute, liquid
27	2.5	Cream substitute, light, liquid
27	14.8	Cream substitute, powdered
27	19.8	Cream substitute, light, powdered
55	12.8	Whipped topping, nondairy
55	8.9	Whipped topping, nondairy, pressurized can
55	12.8	Whipped topping, nondairy, frozen
55	13.1	Whipped topping, nondairy, frozen, lowfat
55	9.2	Whipped cream substitute, nondairy, made from powdered mix
55	5.9	Whipped cream substitute, nondairy, lowfat, low sugar, made from powdered mix
27	1.2	Sour cream
27	1.2	Sour cream, half and half
27	1.9	Sour cream, reduced fat
27	1.9	Sour cream, light
32	5.0	Sour cream, fat free
27	2.3	Dip, sour cream base
27	2.3	Dip, sour cream base, reduced calorie

GI	GL	Food Name
27	1.7	Spinach dip, sour cream base

Milk Desserts, Sauces, Gravies

GI	GL	Food Name
61	14.9	Ice cream
61	14.4	Ice cream, regular, flavors other than chocolate
61	17.2	Ice cream, regular, chocolate
38	8.5	Ice cream, rich, flavors other than chocolate
37	7.7	Ice cream, rich, chocolate
37	8.2	Ice cream, rich
61	14.4	Ice cream, soft serve, flavors other than chocolate
61	17.0	Ice cream, soft serve, chocolate
61	13.5	Ice cream, soft serve
61	14.4	Ice cream bar or stick, not chocolate covered or cake covered
61	15.6	Ice cream bar or stick, chocolate covered
61	17.7	Ice cream bar or stick, chocolate or caramel covered, with nuts
61	21.4	Ice cream bar or stick, rich chocolate ice cream, thick chocolate covering
61	20.4	Ice cream bar or stick, rich ice cream, thick chocolate covering
61	18.0	Ice cream bar or stick, rich ice cream, chocolate covered, with nuts
61	21.3	Ice cream bar or stick, chocolate ice cream, chocolate covered
65	9.0	Ice cream soda, flavors other than chocolate
60	9.1	Ice cream soda, chocolate
50	12.9	Light ice cream

MILK and MILK PRODUCTS

GI	GL	Food Name
50	12.9	Light ice cream, flavors other than chocolate
50	12.9	Light ice cream, chocolate
50	10.9	Light ice cream, soft serve
50	10.9	Light ice cream, soft serve, flavors other than chocolate
50	12.9	Light ice cream, soft serve, chocolate
50	11.7	Light ice cream, soft serve cone, flavors other than chocolate
50	12.7	Light ice cream, soft serve cone, chocolate
50	11.7	Light ice cream, soft serve cone
50	13.7	Light ice cream, bar or stick, chocolate-coated
50	14.0	Light ice cream, cone
50	13.1	Light ice cream, cone, flavors other than chocolate
50	15.0	Light ice cream, cone, chocolate
50	14.1	Light ice cream, creamsicle or dreamsicle
50	13.5	Light ice cream, fudgesicle
42	12.8	Sherbet, all flavors
42	10.2	Fat free ice cream, no sugar added, chocolate
42	10.6	Fat free ice cream, no sugar added, flavors other than chocolate
42	12.6	Fat free ice cream, flavors other than chocolate
42	15.8	Fat free ice cream, chocolate
42	12.6	Fat free ice cream
44	8.5	Pudding
62	14.3	Pudding, bread

GI	GL	Food Name
44	8.3	Pudding, chocolate, ready-to-eat
44	6.7	Pudding, chocolate, ready-to-eat, low calorie, containing artificial sweetener
44	8.2	Pudding, flavors other than chocolate, ready-to-eat
44	7.1	Pudding, flavors other than chocolate, ready-to-eat, low calorie, containing artificial sweetener
38	4.1	Custard
38	10.3	Custard, Puerto Rican style (Flan)
54	14.4	Pudding, rice
54	13.5	Pudding, rice flour, with nuts (Indian dessert)
63	10.6	Pudding, tapioca, made with milk
63	12.3	Pudding, tapioca, made from dry mix, made with milk
63	13.2	Pudding, tapioca, chocolate, made with milk
44	7.8	Pudding, coconut
44	9.1	Pudding, Indian (milk, molasses and cornmeal-based pudding)
44	7.2	Pudding, pumpkin
44	8.5	Pudding, flavors other than chocolate, prepared from dry mix, milk added
44	8.4	Pudding, chocolate, prepared from dry mix, milk added
44	4.2	Pudding, flavors other than chocolate, prepared from dry mix, low calorie, containing artificial sweetener, milk added
44	4.5	Pudding, chocolate, prepared from dry mix, low calorie, containing artificial sweetener, milk added
44	8.9	Pudding, canned, chocolate, reduced fat

MILK and MILK PRODUCTS

GI	GL	Food Name
44	8.9	Pudding, canned, chocolate, fat free
44	10.0	Pudding, canned, flavors other than chocolate, reduced fat
44	10.0	Pudding, canned, flavors other than chocolate, fat free
44	9.7	Pudding, canned, flavors other than chocolate
44	10.0	Pudding, canned, low calorie, containing artificial sweetener, flavors other than chocolate
44	10.1	Pudding, canned, chocolate
44	8.9	Pudding, canned, low calorie, containing artificial sweetener, chocolate
44	9.9	Pudding, canned, chocolate and non-chocolate flavors combined
63	12.1	Pudding, canned, tapioca
63	12.8	Pudding, canned, tapioca, fat free
59	15.5	Pudding, with fruit and vanilla wafers
34	5.5	Mousse, chocolate
34	5.7	Mousse, not chocolate
38	15.2	Coconut custard, Puerto Rican style (Flan de coco)
27	2.5	White sauce, milk sauce
50	4.2	Milk gravy, quick gravy

Cheeses

GI	GL	Food Name
27	1.3	Cheese
27	1.4	Cheese, Cheddar or American type, NS as to natural or processed
27	0.7	Cheese, natural
27	0.6	Cheese, Blue or Roquefort

GI	GL	Food Name
27	0.8	Cheese, Brick
27	0.1	Cheese, Camembert
27	0.1	Cheese, Brie
27	0.3	Cheese, natural, Cheddar or American type
27	0.5	Cheese, Cheddar or American type, dry, grated
27	0.7	Cheese, Colby
27	0.4	Cheese, Colby Jack
27	1.1	Cheese, Feta
27	0.4	Cheese, Fontina
27	0.5	Cheese, goat
27	0.5	Cheese, Gouda or Edam
27	0.1	Cheese, Gruyere
27	0.1	Cheese, Limburger
27	0.2	Cheese, Monterey
27	0.2	Cheese, Monterey, lowfat
27	1.0	Cheese, Mozzarella
27	0.6	Cheese, Mozzarella, whole milk
27	1.0	Cheese, Mozzarella, part skim
27	0.8	Cheese, Mozzarella, low sodium
32	1.1	Cheese, Mozzarella, nonfat or fat free
27	0.3	Cheese, Muenster
27	0.9	Cheese, Muenster, lowfat
27	1.1	Cheese, Parmesan, dry grated
27	0.9	Cheese, Parmesan, hard

MILK and MILK PRODUCTS

GI	GL	Food Name
27	1.0	Cheese, Parmesan, low sodium
32	12.8	Parmesan cheese topping, fat free
27	0.2	Cheese, Port du Salut
27	0.6	Cheese, Provolone
27	1.5	Cheese, Swiss
27	0.9	Cheese, Swiss, low sodium
27	0.9	Cheese, Swiss, lowfat
27	0.5	Cheese, Cheddar or Colby, low sodium
27	0.5	Cheese, Cheddar or Colby, lowfat
27	0.5	Cheese, Mexican blend
27	1.3	Queso Anejo (aged Mexican cheese)
27	0.8	Queso Asadero
27	1.5	Queso Chihuahua
27	1.5	Queso Fresco
30	0.8	Cheese, cottage
27	0.7	Cheese, cottage, creamed, large or small curd
27	0.7	Cottage cheese, farmer's
27	1.1	Cheese, Ricotta
43	2.0	Cheese, cottage, with fruit
27	0.5	Cheese, cottage, dry curd
32	0.6	Cheese, cottage, salted, dry curd
27	0.8	Puerto Rican white cheese (queso del pais, blanco)
32	0.9	Cheese, cottage, lowfat (1-2% fat)
45	3.4	Cheese, cottage, lowfat, with fruit

GI	GL	Food Name
32	1.0	Cheese, cottage, lowfat, with vegetables
32	0.9	Cheese, cottage, lowfat, low sodium
27	0.9	Cheese, cottage, lowfat, lactose reduced
27	0.7	Cheese, cream
27	1.9	Cheese, cream, light or lite (formerly called Cream Cheese Lowfat)
27	0.4	Cheese, processed, American and Swiss blends
27	1.9	Cheese, processed, American or Cheddar type
27	0.4	Cheese, processed, American or Cheddar type, low sodium
27	0.9	Cheese, processed, American or Cheddar type, lowfat
27	2.9	Cheese, processed cheese product, American or Cheddar type, reduced fat
32	4.3	Cheese, processed, American or Cheddar type, nonfat or fat free
32	1.9	Cheese, processed cream cheese product, nonfat or fat free
27	0.6	Cheese, processed, Swiss
27	1.2	Cheese, processed, Swiss, lowfat
27	2.1	Cheese, processed cheese food
27	0.5	Cheese, processed, with vegetables
27	2.1	Cheese, processed, with wine
27	2.4	Cheese spread
27	2.4	Cheese spread, American or Cheddar cheese base
27	2.4	Cheese spread, Swiss cheese base

MILK and MILK PRODUCTS

GI	GL	Food Name
27	0.9	Cheese spread, cream cheese, regular
27	2.4	Cheese spread, pressurized can
27	3.1	Imitation cheese, American or cheddar type
27	0.3	Imitation cheese, American or cheddar type, low cholesterol
27	6.4	Imitation mozzarella cheese
43	3.4	Cheese, cottage cheese, with gelatin dessert
43	5.5	Cheese, cottage cheese, with gelatin dessert and fruit
43	2.5	Cheese, cottage cheese, with gelatin dessert and vegetables
27	1.0	Cheese with nuts
27	0.9	Dip, cream cheese base
27	0.9	Shrimp dip, cream cheese base
27	2.0	Dip, cheese with chili pepper (chili con queso)
27	2.4	Dip, cheese base other than cream cheese
27	1.6	Welsh rarebit
27	2.0	Cheese sauce
27	1.8	Cheese sauce made with lowfat cheese
27	0.7	Alfredo sauce
27	4.1	Cheese, nuggets or pieces, breaded, baked, or fried
27	1.8	Cheddar cheese soup

MEAT, POULTRY, FISH and MIXTURES

Beef

GI	GL	Food Name
0	0.0	Ground meat
0	0.0	Beef, cooked
0	0.0	Beef, cooked, lean and fat eaten
0	0.0	Beef, cooked, lean only eaten
0	0.0	Steak, cooked
0	0.0	Steak, cooked, lean and fat eaten
0	0.0	Steak, cooked, lean only eaten
50	0.2	Beef, pickled
0	0.0	Beef steak
0	0.0	Beef steak, lean and fat eaten
0	0.0	Beef steak, lean only eaten
0	0.0	Beef steak, broiled or baked
0	0.0	Beef steak, broiled or baked, lean and fat eaten
0	0.0	Beef steak, broiled or baked, lean only eaten
0	0.0	Beef steak, fried
0	0.0	Beef steak, fried, lean and fat eaten
0	0.0	Beef steak, fried, lean only eaten
50	5.5	Beef steak, breaded or floured, baked or fried
50	5.5	Beef steak, breaded or floured, baked or fried, lean and fat eaten
50	5.5	Beef steak, breaded or floured, baked or fried, lean only eaten
50	3.6	Beef steak, battered, fried

MEAT, POULTRY, FISH and MIXTURES

GI	GL	Food Name
50	3.6	Beef steak, battered, fried, lean and fat eaten
50	3.6	Beef steak, battered, fried, lean only eaten
0	0.0	Beef steak, braised
0	0.0	Beef steak, braised, lean and fat eaten
0	0.0	Beef steak, braised, lean only eaten
0	0.0	Beef, oxtails, cooked
0	0.0	Beef, neck bones, cooked
0	0.0	Beef, shortribs, cooked
0	0.0	Beef, shortribs, cooked, lean and fat eaten
0	0.0	Beef, shortribs, cooked, lean only eaten
50	1.8	Beef, shortribs, barbecued, with sauce
50	1.8	Beef, shortribs, barbecued, with sauce, lean and fat
50	2.9	Beef, shortribs, barbecued, with sauce, lean only eaten
0	0.0	Beef, cow head, cooked
0	0.0	Beef, roast, roasted
0	0.0	Beef, roast, roasted, lean and fat eaten
0	0.0	Beef, roast, roasted, lean only eaten
0	0.0	Beef, roast, canned
0	0.0	Beef, pot roast, braised or boiled
0	0.0	Beef, pot roast, braised or boiled, lean and fat eaten
0	0.0	Beef, pot roast, braised or boiled, lean only eaten
0	0.0	Beef, stew meat, cooked
0	0.0	Beef, stew meat, cooked, lean and fat eaten
0	0.0	Beef, stew meat, cooked, lean only eaten

GI	GL	Food Name
50	0.2	Corned beef, cooked
50	0.2	Corned beef, cooked, lean and fat eaten
0	0.0	Corned beef, cooked, lean only eaten
0	0.0	Corned beef, canned, ready-to-eat
0	0.0	Beef brisket, cooked
0	0.0	Beef brisket, cooked, lean and fat eaten
0	0.0	Beef brisket, cooked, lean only eaten
0	0.0	Beef, sandwich steak (flaked, formed, thinly sliced)
0	0.0	Ground beef, raw
0	0.0	Ground beef or patty, cooked
0	0.0	Ground beef, meatballs, meat only, cooked
95	14.2	Ground beef or patty, breaded, cooked
0	0.0	Ground beef, regular, cooked
0	0.0	Ground beef, lean, cooked
0	0.0	Ground beef, extra lean, cooked
50	0.7	Beef, bacon, cooked
50	2.9	Beef, bacon, cooked, lean only eaten
50	0.7	Beef, bacon, formed, lean meat added, cooked
50	1.4	Beef, dried, chipped, uncooked
0	0.0	Beef, dried, chipped, cooked in fat
50	0.0	Beef, pastrami (beef, smoked, spiced)
0	0.0	Beef, baby food
0	0.0	Beef, baby food, strained
0	0.0	Beef, baby food, junior

GI	GL	Food Name

Pork

GI	GL	Food Name
0	0.0	Pork, cooked
0	0.0	Pork, cooked, lean and fat eaten
0	0.0	Pork, cooked, lean only eaten
0	0.0	Pork, fried
0	0.0	Pork, fried, lean and fat eaten
0	0.0	Pork, fried, lean only eaten
0	0.0	Pork, ground or patty, cooked
95	14.2	Pork, ground or patty, breaded, cooked
0	0.0	Pork chop
0	0.0	Pork chop, lean and fat eaten
0	0.0	Pork chop, lean only eaten
0	0.0	Pork chop, broiled or baked
0	0.0	Pork chop, broiled or baked, lean and fat eaten
0	0.0	Pork chop, broiled or baked, lean only eaten
95	7.4	Pork chop, breaded or floured, broiled or baked
95	7.4	Pork chop, breaded or floured, broiled or baked, lean and fat eaten
95	7.4	Pork chop, breaded or floured, broiled or baked, lean only eaten
0	0.0	Pork chop, fried
0	0.0	Pork chop, fried, lean and fat eaten
0	0.0	Pork chop, fried, lean only eaten
95	13.1	Pork chop, breaded or floured, fried
95	13.1	Pork chop, breaded or floured, fried, lean and fat eaten

GI	GL	Food Name
95	13.5	Pork chop, breaded or floured, fried, lean only eaten
95	6.2	Pork chop, battered, fried
95	6.2	Pork chop, battered, fried, lean and fat eaten
95	6.1	Pork chop, battered, fried, lean only eaten
0	0.0	Pork chop, stewed
0	0.0	Pork chop, stewed, lean and fat eaten
0	0.0	Pork chop, stewed, lean only eaten
0	0.0	Pork chop, smoked or cured, cooked
0	0.0	Pork chop, smoked or cured, cooked, lean and fat eaten
0	0.0	Pork chop, smoked or cured, cooked, lean only eaten
0	0.0	Pork steak or cutlet
0	0.0	Pork steak or cutlet, lean and fat eaten
0	0.0	Pork steak or cutlet, lean only eaten
95	6.2	Pork steak or cutlet, battered, fried
95	6.3	Pork steak or cutlet, battered, fried, lean and fat eaten
95	6.2	Pork steak or cutlet, battered, fried, lean only eaten
0	0.0	Pork steak or cutlet, broiled or baked
0	0.0	Pork steak or cutlet, broiled or baked, lean and fat eaten
0	0.0	Pork steak or cutlet, broiled or baked, lean only eaten
0	0.0	Pork steak or cutlet, fried
0	0.0	Pork steak or cutlet, fried, lean and fat eaten
0	0.0	Pork steak or cutlet, fried, lean only eaten
95	7.1	Pork steak or cutlet, breaded or floured, broiled or baked

MEAT, POULTRY, FISH and MIXTURES

GI	GL	Food Name
95	7.1	Pork steak or cutlet, breaded or floured, broiled or baked, lean and fat eaten
95	7.1	Pork steak or cutlet, breaded or floured, broiled or baked, lean only eaten
95	8.9	Pork steak or cutlet, breaded or floured, fried
95	8.9	Pork steak or cutlet, breaded or floured, fried, lean and fat eaten
95	9.2	Pork steak or cutlet, breaded or floured, fried, lean only eaten
0	0.0	Pork, tenderloin, cooked
95	7.0	Pork, tenderloin, breaded, fried
0	0.0	Pork, tenderloin, braised
0	0.0	Pork, tenderloin, baked
95	6.6	Pork, tenderloin, battered, fried
50	0.2	Ham, fried
50	0.2	Ham, fried, lean and fat eaten
0	0.0	Ham, fried, lean only eaten
95	6.2	Ham, breaded or floured, fried
95	6.2	Ham, breaded or floured, fried, lean and fat eaten
95	5.6	Ham, breaded or floured, fried, lean only eaten
0	0.0	Ham, fresh, cooked
0	0.0	Ham, fresh, cooked, lean and fat eaten
0	0.0	Ham, fresh, cooked, lean only eaten
50	0.1	Ham, smoked or cured, cooked
50	0.1	Ham, smoked or cured, cooked, lean and fat eaten

GI	GL	Food Name
0	0.0	Ham, smoked or cured, cooked, lean only eaten
50	0.3	Ham, smoked or cured, low sodium, cooked
50	0.2	Ham, smoked or cured, low sodium, cooked, lean and fat eaten
50	0.2	Ham, prosciutto
0	0.0	Ham, smoked or cured, canned
50	0.0	Ham, smoked or cured, canned, lean and fat eaten
0	0.0	Ham, smoked or cured, canned, lean only eaten
50	0.9	Ham, smoked or cured, ground patty
0	0.0	Pork roast, cooked
0	0.0	Pork roast, cooked, lean and fat eaten
0	0.0	Pork roast, cooked, lean only eaten
0	0.0	Pork roast, loin, cooked
0	0.0	Pork roast, loin, cooked, lean and fat eaten
0	0.0	Pork roast, loin, cooked, lean only eaten
0	0.0	Pork roast, shoulder, cooked
0	0.0	Pork roast, shoulder, cooked, lean and fat eaten
0	0.0	Pork roast, shoulder, cooked, lean only eaten
50	0.3	Pork roast, smoked or cured, cooked
50	0.3	Pork roast, smoked or cured, cooked, lean and fat eaten
0	0.0	Pork roast, smoked or cured, cooked, lean only eaten
28	0.5	Pork roll, cured, fried
50	0.7	Canadian bacon, cooked
50	0.7	Bacon, cooked

GI	GL	Food Name
50	0.7	Pork bacon, NS as to fresh, smoked or cured, cooked
50	0.7	Pork bacon, smoked or cured, cooked
50	0.7	Pork bacon, smoked or cured, cooked, lean only eaten
50	0.7	Bacon or side pork, fresh, cooked
50	0.7	Pork bacon, smoked or cured, lower sodium
50	0.5	Pork bacon, formed, lean meat added, cooked
0	0.0	Salt pork, cooked
0	0.0	Fat back, cooked
0	0.0	Pork, spareribs, cooked
0	0.0	Pork, spareribs, cooked, lean and fat eaten
0	0.0	Pork, spareribs, cooked, lean only eaten
50	2.1	Pork, spareribs, barbecued, with sauce
50	2.1	Pork, spareribs, barbecued, with sauce, lean and fat
50	2.1	Pork, spareribs, barbecued, with sauce, lean only eaten
50	0.0	Pork ears, tail, head, snout, miscellaneous parts, cooked
0	0.0	Pork, neck bones, cooked
0	0.0	Pork, pig's feet, cooked
32	0.1	Pork, pig's feet, pickled
0	0.0	Pork, pig's hocks, cooked
0	0.0	Pork skin, rinds, deep-fried
0	0.0	Pork skin, boiled

Lamb, Veal, Game

0	0.0	Lamb, cooked
0	0.0	Lamb chop, cooked

GI	GL	Food Name
0	0.0	Lamb chop, cooked, lean and fat eaten
0	0.0	Lamb chop, cooked, lean only eaten
0	0.0	Lamb, loin chop, cooked
0	0.0	Lamb, loin chop, cooked, lean and fat eaten
0	0.0	Lamb, loin chop, cooked, lean only eaten
0	0.0	Lamb, shoulder chop, cooked
0	0.0	Lamb, shoulder chop, cooked, lean and fat eaten
0	0.0	Lamb, shoulder chop, cooked, lean only eaten
0	0.0	Lamb, shoulder, cooked
0	0.0	Lamb, shoulder, cooked, lean and fat eaten
0	0.0	Lamb, shoulder, cooked, lean only eaten
0	0.0	Lamb, ribs, cooked, lean only eaten
0	0.0	Lamb, ribs, cooked
0	0.0	Lamb, ribs, cooked, lean and fat eaten
0	0.0	Lamb hocks, cooked
0	0.0	Lamb, roast, cooked
0	0.0	Lamb, roast, cooked, lean and fat eaten
0	0.0	Lamb, roast, cooked, lean only eaten
0	0.0	Lamb, ground or patty, cooked
0	0.0	Goat, boiled
0	0.0	Goat, fried
0	0.0	Goat, baked
0	0.0	Goat ribs, cooked
0	0.0	Veal, cooked

MEAT, POULTRY, FISH and MIXTURES

GI	GL	Food Name
0	0.0	Veal, cooked, lean and fat eaten
0	0.0	Veal, cooked, lean only eaten
0	0.0	Veal chop
0	0.0	Veal chop, lean and fat eaten
0	0.0	Veal chop, lean only eaten
50	4.3	Veal chop, fried
50	4.9	Veal chop, fried, lean and fat eaten
50	4.3	Veal chop, fried, lean only eaten
0	0.0	Veal chop, broiled
0	0.0	Veal chop, broiled, lean and fat eaten
0	0.0	Veal chop, broiled, lean only eaten
0	0.0	Veal cutlet or steak
0	0.0	Veal cutlet or steak, lean and fat eaten
0	0.0	Veal cutlet or steak, lean only eaten
0	0.0	Veal cutlet or steak, broiled
0	0.0	Veal cutlet or steak, broiled, lean and fat eaten
0	0.0	Veal cutlet or steak, broiled, lean only eaten
50	4.9	Veal cutlet or steak, fried
50	4.9	Veal cutlet or steak, fried, lean and fat eaten
0	0.0	Veal cutlet or steak, fried, lean only eaten
0	0.0	Veal, roasted
0	0.0	Veal, roasted, lean and fat eaten
0	0.0	Veal, roasted, lean only eaten
0	0.0	Veal, ground or patty, cooked

GI	GL	Food Name
50	4.2	Veal patty, breaded, cooked
0	0.0	Rabbit, NS as to domestic or wild, cooked
0	0.0	Rabbit, domestic
0	0.0	Rabbit, wild, cooked
0	0.0	Venison/deer
0	0.0	Venison/deer, cured
0	0.0	Venison/deer, roasted
0	0.0	Venison/deer steak, cooked
50	6.2	Venison/deer steak, breaded or floured, cooked
50	7.4	Venison/deer jerky
28	1.1	Deer bologna
0	0.0	Deer chop, cooked
0	0.0	Venison/deer ribs, cooked
0	0.0	Venison/deer, stewed
0	0.0	Moose, cooked
0	0.0	Bear, cooked
0	0.0	Caribou, cooked
0	0.0	Bison, cooked
0	0.0	Ground hog, cooked
0	0.0	Opossum, cooked
0	0.0	Squirrel, cooked
0	0.0	Beaver, cooked
0	0.0	Raccoon, cooked
0	0.0	Armadillo, cooked

GI	GL	Food Name
0	0.0	Wild pig, smoked
0	0.0	Ostrich, cooked

Poultry

GI	GL	Food Name
0	0.0	Chicken
0	0.0	Chicken, skin eaten
0	0.0	Chicken, skin not eaten
0	0.0	Chicken, roasted, broiled, or baked
0	0.0	Chicken, roasted, broiled, or baked, skin eaten
0	0.0	Chicken, roasted, broiled, or baked, skin not eaten
0	0.0	Chicken, stewed
0	0.0	Chicken, stewed, skin eaten
0	0.0	Chicken, stewed, skin not eaten
0	0.0	Chicken, fried, no coating
0	0.0	Chicken, fried, no coating, skin eaten
0	0.0	Chicken, fried, no coating, skin not eaten
95	9.5	Chicken, coated, baked or fried, prepared with skin
95	9.5	Chicken, coated, baked or fried, prepared with skin, skin/coating eaten
0	0.0	Chicken, coated, baked or fried, prepared with skin, skin/coating not eaten
0	0.0	Chicken, coated, baked or fried, prepared skinless, coating not eaten
0	0.0	Chicken, breast
0	0.0	Chicken, breast, skin eaten

GI	GL	Food Name
0	0.0	Chicken, breast, skin not eaten
0	0.0	Chicken, breast, roasted, broiled, or baked
0	0.0	Chicken, breast, roasted, broiled, or baked, skin eaten
0	0.0	Chicken, breast, roasted, broiled, or baked, skin not
0	0.0	Chicken, breast, stewed
0	0.0	Chicken, breast, stewed, skin eaten
0	0.0	Chicken, breast, stewed, skin not eaten
0	0.0	Chicken, breast, fried, no coating
0	0.0	Chicken, breast, fried, no coating, skin eaten
0	0.0	Chicken, breast, fried, no coating, skin not eaten
95	9.0	Chicken, breast, coated, baked or fried, prepared with
95	9.0	Chicken, breast, coated, baked or fried, prepared with skin, skin/coating eaten
95	0.0	Chicken, breast, coated, baked or fried, prepared with skin, skin/coating not eaten
95	9.2	Chicken, breast, coated, baked or fried, prepared
95	9.2	Chicken, breast, coated, baked or fried, prepared skinless, coating eaten
95	0.0	Chicken, breast, coated, baked or fried, prepared skinless, coating not eaten
0	0.0	Chicken, leg (drumstick and thigh)
0	0.0	Chicken, leg (drumstick and thigh), skin eaten
0	0.0	Chicken, leg (drumstick and thigh), skin not eaten
0	0.0	Chicken, leg (drumstick and thigh), roasted, broiled, or baked

MEAT, POULTRY, FISH and MIXTURES

GI	GL	Food Name
0	0.0	Chicken, leg (drumstick and thigh), roasted, broiled, or baked, skin eaten
0	0.0	Chicken, leg (drumstick and thigh), roasted, broiled, or baked, skin not eaten
0	0.0	Chicken, leg (drumstick and thigh), stewed
0	0.0	Chicken, leg (drumstick and thigh), stewed, skin eaten
0	0.0	Chicken, leg (drumstick and thigh), stewed, skin not
0	0.0	Chicken, leg (drumstick and thigh), fried, no coating
0	0.0	Chicken, leg (drumstick and thigh), fried, no coating, skin eaten
0	0.0	Chicken, leg (drumstick and thigh), fried, no coating, skin not eaten
95	8.3	Chicken, leg (drumstick and thigh), coated, baked or fried, prepared with skin
95	8.3	Chicken, leg (drumstick and thigh), coated, baked or fried, prepared with skin, skin/coating eaten
95	0.0	Chicken, leg (drumstick and thigh), coated, baked or fried, prepared with skin, skin/coating not eaten
95	9.6	Chicken, leg (drumstick and thigh), coated, baked or fried, prepared skinless
95	9.6	Chicken, leg (drumstick and thigh), coated, baked or fried, prepared skinless, coating eaten
95	0.0	Chicken, leg (drumstick and thigh), coated, baked or fried, prepared skinless, coating not eaten
0	0.0	Chicken, drumstick
0	0.0	Chicken, drumstick, skin eaten
0	0.0	Chicken, drumstick, skin not eaten

GI	GL	Food Name
0	0.0	Chicken, drumstick, roasted, broiled, or baked
0	0.0	Chicken, drumstick, roasted, broiled, or baked, skin
0	0.0	Chicken, drumstick, roasted, broiled, or baked, skin not eaten
0	0.0	Chicken, drumstick, stewed
0	0.0	Chicken, drumstick, stewed, skin eaten
0	0.0	Chicken, drumstick, stewed, skin not eaten
0	0.0	Chicken, drumstick, fried, no coating
0	0.0	Chicken, drumstick, fried, no coating, skin eaten
0	0.0	Chicken, drumstick, fried, no coating, skin not eaten
95	7.8	Chicken, drumstick, coated, baked or fried, prepared with skin
95	7.8	Chicken, drumstick, coated, baked or fried, prepared with skin, skin/coating eaten
0	0.0	Chicken, drumstick, coated, baked or fried, prepared with skin, skin/coating not eaten
95	7.6	Chicken, drumstick, coated, baked or fried, prepared skinless
95	7.6	Chicken, drumstick, coated, baked or fried, prepared skinless, coating eaten
0	0.0	Chicken, drumstick, coated, baked or fried, prepared skinless, coating not eaten
0	0.0	Chicken, thigh
0	0.0	Chicken, thigh, skin eaten
0	0.0	Chicken, thigh, skin not eaten
0	0.0	Chicken, thigh, roasted, broiled, or baked

MEAT, POULTRY, FISH and MIXTURES

GI	GL	Food Name
0	0.0	Chicken, thigh, roasted, broiled, or baked, skin eaten
0	0.0	Chicken, thigh, roasted, broiled, or baked, skin not eaten
0	0.0	Chicken, thigh, stewed
0	0.0	Chicken, thigh, stewed, skin eaten
0	0.0	Chicken, thigh, stewed, skin not eaten
0	0.0	Chicken, thigh, fried, no coating
0	0.0	Chicken, thigh, fried, no coating, skin eaten
0	0.0	Chicken, thigh, fried, no coating, skin not eaten
95	9.4	Chicken, thigh, coated, baked or fried, prepared with skin
95	9.4	Chicken, thigh, coated, baked or fried, prepared with skin, skin/coating eaten
95	0.0	Chicken, thigh, coated, baked or fried, prepared with skin, skin/coating not eaten
95	9.7	Chicken, thigh, coated, baked or fried, prepared skinless
95	9.7	Chicken, thigh, coated, baked or fried, prepared skinless, coating eaten
95	0.0	Chicken, thigh, coated, baked or fried, prepared skinless, coating not eaten
0	0.0	Chicken, wing
0	0.0	Chicken, wing, skin eaten
0	0.0	Chicken, wing, skin not eaten
0	0.0	Chicken, wing, roasted, broiled, or baked
0	0.0	Chicken, wing, roasted, broiled, or baked, skin eaten
0	0.0	Chicken, wing, roasted, broiled, or baked, skin not eaten
0	0.0	Chicken, wing, stewed

GI	GL	Food Name
0	0.0	Chicken, wing, stewed, skin eaten
0	0.0	Chicken, wing, stewed, skin not eaten
0	0.0	Chicken, wing, fried, no coating
0	0.0	Chicken, wing, fried, no coating, skin eaten
0	0.0	Chicken, wing, fried, no coating, skin not eaten
95	10.5	Chicken, wing, coated, baked or fried, prepared with skin
95	10.5	Chicken, wing, coated, baked or fried, prepared with skin, skin/coating eaten
0	0.0	Chicken, wing, coated, baked or fried, prepared with skin, skin/coating not eaten
0	0.0	Chicken, back
0	0.0	Chicken, neck or ribs
0	0.0	Chicken skin
50	0.4	Chicken, canned, meat only
0	0.0	Chicken, chicken roll, roasted
95	15.5	Chicken patty, fillet, or tenders, breaded, cooked
0	0.0	Chicken, ground
95	15.5	Chicken nuggets
0	0.0	Turkey
0	0.0	Turkey, light meat, cooked
0	0.0	Turkey, light meat, cooked, skin not eaten
0	0.0	Turkey, light meat, cooked, skin eaten
95	6.1	Turkey, light meat, breaded, baked or fried
95	1.8	Turkey, light meat, breaded, baked or fried, skin not

MEAT, POULTRY, FISH and MIXTURES

GI	GL	Food Name
95	6.1	Turkey, light meat, breaded, baked or fried, skin eaten
0	0.0	Turkey, light meat, roasted
0	0.0	Turkey, light meat, roasted, skin not eaten
0	0.0	Turkey, light meat, roasted, skin eaten
0	0.0	Turkey, dark meat, roasted
0	0.0	Turkey, dark meat, roasted, skin not eaten
0	0.0	Turkey, dark meat, roasted, skin eaten
0	0.0	Turkey, light and dark meat, roasted
0	0.0	Turkey, light and dark meat, roasted, skin not eaten
0	0.0	Turkey, light and dark meat, roasted, skin eaten
0	0.0	Turkey, light or dark meat, stewed
0	0.0	Turkey, light or dark meat, stewed, skin not eaten
0	0.0	Turkey light or dark meat, stewed, skin eaten
0	0.0	Turkey, light or dark meat, smoked, cooked
0	0.0	Turkey, light or dark meat, smoked, cooked, skin eaten
0	0.0	Turkey, light or dark meat, smoked, cooked, skin not eaten
0	0.0	Turkey, drumstick, cooked
0	0.0	Turkey, drumstick, cooked, skin not eaten
0	0.0	Turkey, drumstick, cooked, skin eaten
0	0.0	Turkey, drumstick, roasted
0	0.0	Turkey, drumstick, roasted, skin not eaten
0	0.0	Turkey, drumstick, roasted, skin eaten
0	0.0	Turkey, drumstick, smoked, cooked, skin eaten

GI	GL	Food Name
0	0.0	Turkey, thigh, cooked
0	0.0	Turkey, thigh, cooked, skin eaten
0	0.0	Turkey, thigh, cooked, skin not eaten
0	0.0	Turkey, neck, cooked
0	0.0	Turkey, wing, cooked
0	0.0	Turkey, wing, cooked, skin not eaten
0	0.0	Turkey, wing, cooked, skin eaten
0	0.0	Turkey, wing, smoked, cooked, skin eaten
50	1.5	Turkey, rolled roast, light or dark meat, cooked
0	0.0	Turkey, tail, cooked
0	0.0	Turkey, back, cooked
0	0.0	Turkey, canned
0	0.0	Turkey, ground
95	16.4	Turkey, nuggets
50	1.6	Turkey bacon, cooked
0	0.0	Duck, cooked
0	0.0	Duck, cooked, skin eaten
0	0.0	Duck, cooked, skin not eaten
0	0.0	Duck, roasted
0	0.0	Duck, roasted, skin eaten
0	0.0	Duck, roasted, skin not eaten
0	0.0	Goose, wild, roasted
0	0.0	Cornish game hen, cooked
0	0.0	Cornish game hen, cooked, skin eaten

GI	GL	Food Name
0	0.0	Cornish game hen, cooked, skin not eaten
0	0.0	Cornish game hen, roasted
0	0.0	Cornish game hen, roasted, skin eaten
0	0.0	Cornish game hen, roasted, skin not eaten
0	0.0	Dove, cooked
95	1.4	Dove, fried
0	0.0	Quail, cooked
0	0.0	Pheasant, cooked
50	0.7	Chicken, baby food, strained
50	0.0	Turkey, baby food
50	0.1	Turkey, baby food, strained

Organ Meats, Sausages and Lunchmeats

GI	GL	Food Name
50	2.5	Beef liver, braised
50	2.6	Beef liver, fried
50	0.4	Chicken liver, braised
95	7.4	Chicken liver, fried
50	3.3	Liver paste or pate, chicken
0	0.0	Kidney, cooked
0	0.0	Sweetbreads, cooked
0	0.0	Tongue, cooked
0	0.0	Tripe, cooked
0	0.0	Chitterlings, cooked
0	0.0	Hog maws (stomach), cooked

GI	GL	Food Name
0	0.0	Gizzard, cooked
28	1.2	Frankfurter, wiener, or hot dog
28	1.2	Frankfurter or hot dog, beef
28	0.5	Frankfurter or hot dog, beef and pork
28	1.3	Frankfurter or hot dog, beef and pork, lowfat
28	3.1	Frankfurter or hot dog, meat and poultry, fat free
28	1.2	Frankfurter or hot dog, meat and poultry
28	2.0	Frankfurter or hot dog, chicken
28	0.4	Frankfurter or hot dog, turkey
28	0.5	Frankfurter or hot dog, low salt
28	0.5	Frankfurter or hot dog, beef, lowfat
28	2.4	Frankfurter or hot dog, meat & poultry, lowfat
28	1.0	Cold cut
28	1.1	Beef sausage
28	1.2	Beef sausage, brown and serve, links, cooked
28	1.7	Beef sausage, smoked, stick
28	1.1	Beef sausage, smoked
28	0.5	Beef sausage, fresh, bulk, patty or link, cooked
28	0.4	Blood sausage
28	0.8	Bratwurst, cooked
28	1.5	Bologna, beef, lowfat
28	0.9	Bologna, pork and beef
28	1.5	Bologna
28	0.1	Bologna, Lebanon

MEAT, POULTRY, FISH and MIXTURES

GI	GL	Food Name
28	1.1	Bologna, beef
28	1.3	Bologna, turkey
28	1.5	Bologna ring, smoked
28	0.2	Bologna, pork
28	0.6	Bologna, beef, lower sodium
28	1.5	Bologna, chicken, beef, and pork
28	0.7	Bologna, beef and pork, lowfat
50	1.3	Capicola
0	0.0	Chicken and beef sausage, smoked
28	0.5	Chorizos
0	0.0	Head cheese
28	0.9	Knockwurst
28	0.9	Mortadella
28	1.1	Pepperoni
28	0.6	Polish sausage
28	1.2	Italian sausage
28	0.0	Sausage (not cold cut)
28	0.0	Pork sausage, fresh, bulk, patty or link, cooked
28	0.0	Pork sausage, brown and serve, cooked
28	0.0	Pork sausage, country style, fresh, cooked
28	0.8	Pork and beef sausage
28	0.8	Pork and beef sausage, brown and serve, cooked
28	0.6	Mettwurst
28	0.6	Salami

GI	GL	Food Name
28	0.6	Salami, soft, cooked
28	1.1	Salami, dry or hard
28	0.5	Salami, beef
28	4.2	Scrapple, cooked
28	0.6	Smoked link sausage, pork
28	0.7	Smoked link sausage, pork and beef
28	0.6	Smoked sausage, pork
28	0.0	Souse
28	0.9	Thuringer
0	0.0	Turkey breakfast sausage, bulk
28	1.3	Turkey sausage, smoked
28	0.2	Turkey and pork sausage, fresh, bulk, patty or link,
28	0.7	Turkey, pork, and beef sausage, reduced fat, smoked
28	3.2	Turkey, pork, and beef sausage, lowfat, smoked
28	0.7	Vienna sausage, canned
28	1.9	Vienna sausage, chicken, canned
28	0.7	Luncheon meat
50	1.1	Ham, sliced, prepackaged or deli, luncheon meat
50	0.3	Ham, sliced, low salt, prepackaged or deli, luncheon
50	1.3	Ham, sliced, extra lean, prepackaged or deli, luncheon meat
50	0.9	Chicken or turkey loaf, prepackaged or deli, luncheon meat
50	1.1	Ham loaf, luncheon meat

MEAT, POULTRY, FISH and MIXTURES

GI	GL	Food Name
50	1.1	Ham, luncheon meat, chopped, minced, pressed, spiced, not canned
50	1.3	Ham, luncheon meat, chopped, minced, pressed, spiced, lowfat, not canned
50	2.3	Ham and pork, luncheon meat, chopped, minced, pressed, spiced, canned
50	0.7	Ham, pork and chicken, luncheon meat, chopped, minced, pressed, spiced, canned
50	1.6	Liverwurst
28	2.5	Luncheon loaf (olive, pickle, or pimiento)
28	1.2	Sandwich loaf, luncheon meat
50	0.8	Turkey ham, sliced, extra lean, prepackaged or deli, luncheon meat
50	1.0	Turkey ham
50	1.8	Turkey pastrami
28	0.1	Turkey salami
0	0.0	Turkey or chicken breast, prepackaged or deli, luncheon meat
50	0.4	Beef, sliced, prepackaged or deli, luncheon meat
0	0.0	Corned beef, pressed
50	1.1	Meat spread or potted meat
50	1.1	Ham, deviled or potted

Fish and Shellfish

0	0.0	Fish, raw
0	0.0	Fish, cooked

GI	GL	Food Name
50	0.2	Fish, baked or broiled
95	8.2	Fish, breaded or battered, baked
95	7.8	Fish, floured or breaded, fried
95	6.4	Fish, battered, fried
0	0.0	Fish, steamed
0	0.0	Fish, dried
0	0.0	Fish, canned
0	0.0	Fish, smoked
95	20.1	Fish stick, patty, or fillet, cooked
95	20.1	Fish stick, patty, or fillet, baked or broiled
95	20.1	Fish stick, patty, or fillet, breaded or battered, baked
95	7.8	Fish stick, patty, or fillet, floured or breaded, fried
95	6.4	Fish stick, patty, or fillet, battered, fried
0	0.0	Anchovy, cooked
0	0.0	Anchovy, canned
0	0.0	Barracuda, steamed or poached
95	11.7	Carp, cooked
50	0.3	Carp, baked or broiled
95	11.7	Carp, floured or breaded, fried
0	0.0	Carp, steamed or poached
0	0.0	Carp, smoked
95	8.1	Catfish, cooked
50	0.2	Catfish, baked or broiled
95	8.2	Catfish, breaded or battered, baked

MEAT, POULTRY, FISH and MIXTURES

GI	GL	Food Name
95	8.1	Catfish, floured or breaded, fried
95	6.4	Catfish, battered, fried
0	0.0	Catfish, steamed or poached
95	7.8	Cod, cooked
50	0.2	Cod, baked or broiled
95	8.2	Cod, breaded or battered, baked
95	7.8	Cod, floured or breaded, fried
95	6.6	Cod, battered, fried
0	0.0	Cod, steamed or poached
0	0.0	Cod, dried, salted
0	0.0	Cod, dried, salted, salt removed in water
0	0.0	Cod, smoked
95	13.6	Croaker, cooked
50	0.4	Croaker, baked or broiled
95	8.2	Croaker, breaded or battered, baked
95	13.8	Croaker, floured or breaded, fried
0	0.0	Croaker, steamed or poached
95	5.5	Eel, cooked
0	0.0	Eel, steamed or poached
0	0.0	Eel, smoked
0	0.0	Flounder, raw
50	0.2	Flounder, cooked
50	0.2	Flounder, baked or broiled
95	8.2	Flounder, breaded or battered, baked

GI	GL	Food Name
95	7.8	Flounder, floured or breaded, fried
95	6.4	Flounder, battered, fried
0	0.0	Flounder, steamed or poached
0	0.0	Flounder, smoked
50	0.2	Haddock, cooked
50	0.2	Haddock, baked or broiled
95	8.2	Haddock, breaded or battered, baked
95	7.8	Haddock, floured or breaded, fried
95	6.6	Haddock, battered, fried
0	0.0	Haddock, steamed or poached
0	0.0	Haddock, smoked
0	0.0	Herring, raw
50	0.3	Herring, baked or broiled
0	0.0	Herring, dried, salted
50	4.8	Herring, pickled
0	0.0	Herring, smoked, kippered
0	0.0	Mackerel, raw
50	0.2	Mackerel, cooked
50	0.2	Mackerel, baked or broiled
0	0.0	Mackerel, salted
95	7.8	Mackerel, floured or breaded, fried
0	0.0	Mackerel, pickled
0	0.0	Mackerel, canned
0	0.0	Mackerel, smoked

MEAT, POULTRY, FISH and MIXTURES

GI	GL	Food Name
0	0.0	Mullet, raw
95	12.0	Mullet, cooked
50	0.3	Mullet, baked or broiled
95	12.0	Mullet, floured or breaded, fried
0	0.0	Mullet, steamed or poached
0	0.0	Ocean perch, raw
50	0.2	Ocean perch, cooked
50	0.2	Ocean perch, baked or broiled
95	8.4	Ocean perch, breaded or battered, baked
95	7.8	Ocean perch, floured or breaded, fried
95	6.4	Ocean perch, battered, fried
0	0.0	Ocean perch, steamed or poached
95	13.2	Perch, cooked
50	0.2	Perch, baked or broiled
95	8.4	Perch, breaded or battered, baked
95	13.2	Perch, floured or breaded, fried
95	6.6	Perch, battered, fried
0	0.0	Perch, steamed or poached
95	7.8	Pike, cooked
50	0.2	Pike, baked or broiled
95	7.8	Pike, floured or breaded, fried
95	6.4	Pike, battered, fried
0	0.0	Pike, steamed or poached
0	0.0	Pompano, raw

GI	GL	Food Name
50	0.3	Pompano, cooked
50	0.3	Pompano, baked or broiled
95	12.0	Pompano, floured or breaded, fried
95	6.4	Pompano, battered, fried
0	0.0	Pompano, steamed or poached
0	0.0	Pompano, smoked
0	0.0	Porgy, raw
95	13.8	Porgy, cooked
50	0.4	Porgy, baked or broiled
95	12.1	Porgy, breaded or battered, baked
95	13.8	Porgy, floured or breaded, fried
95	10.1	Porgy, battered, fried
0	0.0	Porgy, steamed or poached
50	0.2	Ray, cooked
50	0.2	Ray, baked or broiled
95	12.0	Ray, floured or breaded, fried
0	0.0	Ray, steamed or poached
0	0.0	Salmon, raw
0	0.0	Salmon, cooked
50	0.2	Salmon, baked or broiled
95	9.4	Salmon, floured or breaded, fried
95	6.4	Salmon, battered, fried
0	0.0	Salmon, steamed or poached
0	0.0	Salmon, dried

MEAT, POULTRY, FISH and MIXTURES

GI	GL	Food Name
0	0.0	Salmon, canned
0	0.0	Salmon, smoked
0	0.0	Sardines, cooked
0	0.0	Sardines, dried
0	0.0	Sardines, canned in oil
0	0.0	Sardines, skinless, boneless, packed in water
50	0.2	Sea bass, cooked
50	0.2	Sea bass, baked or broiled
95	8.4	Sea bass, breaded or battered, baked
95	9.4	Sea bass, floured or breaded, fried
0	0.0	Sea bass, steamed or poached
50	0.4	Sea bass, pickled (Mero en escabeche)
50	0.2	Shark, cooked
50	0.2	Shark, baked or broiled
0	0.0	Shark, steamed or poached
95	12.0	Smelt, cooked
50	0.3	Smelt, baked or broiled
95	12.0	Smelt, floured or breaded, fried
95	9.0	Smelt, battered, fried
0	0.0	Smelt, steamed or poached
0	0.0	Sturgeon, cooked
0	0.0	Sturgeon, baked or broiled
0	0.0	Sturgeon, steamed
0	0.0	Sturgeon, smoked

GI	GL	Food Name
50	0.2	Swordfish, cooked
50	0.2	Swordfish, baked or broiled
95	7.8	Swordfish, floured or breaded, fried
0	0.0	Swordfish, steamed or poached
50	0.2	Trout, cooked
50	0.2	Trout, baked or broiled
95	8.6	Trout, breaded or battered, baked
95	9.4	Trout, floured or breaded, fried
95	6.6	Trout, battered, fried
0	0.0	Trout, steamed or poached
0	0.0	Trout, smoked
0	0.0	Tuna, fresh, raw
50	0.2	Tuna, fresh, cooked
50	0.2	Tuna, fresh, baked or broiled
95	7.8	Tuna, fresh, floured or breaded, fried
0	0.0	Tuna, fresh, steamed or poached
0	0.0	Tuna, fresh, dried
0	0.0	Tuna, fresh, smoked
0	0.0	Tuna, canned, NS as to oil or water pack
0	0.0	Tuna, canned, oil pack
0	0.0	Tuna, canned, water pack
50	0.2	Whiting, cooked
50	0.2	Whiting, baked or broiled
95	8.2	Whiting, breaded or battered, baked

MEAT, POULTRY, FISH and MIXTURES

GI	GL	Food Name
95	7.8	Whiting, floured or breaded, fried
95	6.6	Whiting, battered, fried
0	0.0	Whiting, steamed or poached
0	0.0	Frog legs, steamed
0	0.0	Jellyfish, pickled
95	10.2	Octopus, cooked
50	2.2	Octopus, steamed
50	2.2	Octopus, dried, boiled
50	1.1	Roe, shad, cooked
50	2.0	Roe, sturgeon
50	1.9	Squid, baked, broiled
95	11.0	Squid, breaded, fried
50	1.8	Squid, steamed or boiled
50	1.5	Squid, pickled
50	1.8	Squid, canned
50	1.3	Clams, raw
95	10.5	Clams, cooked
50	1.6	Clams, baked or broiled
95	10.5	Clams, floured or breaded, fried
95	12.5	Clams, battered, fried
50	1.6	Clams, steamed or boiled
50	1.6	Clams, canned
50	0.9	Conch, baked or broiled
0	0.0	Crab, cooked

GI	GL	Food Name
50	0.1	Crab, baked or broiled
0	0.0	Crab, hard shell, steamed
0	0.0	Crab, canned
95	16.2	Crab, soft shell, floured or breaded, fried
95	10.5	Crayfish, floured or breaded, fried
0	0.0	Crayfish, boiled or steamed
50	0.6	Lobster, cooked
50	0.6	Lobster, baked or broiled
50	0.6	Lobster, without shell, steamed or boiled
50	0.6	Lobster, steamed or boiled
95	4.2	Mussels, cooked
50	3.7	Mussels, steamed or poached
50	2.0	Oysters, raw
95	11.9	Oysters, cooked
50	1.9	Oysters, baked or broiled
50	2.4	Oysters, steamed
95	11.4	Oysters, floured or breaded, fried
95	13.6	Oysters, battered, fried
50	2.1	Oysters, canned
50	3.2	Oysters, smoked
95	10.0	Scallops, cooked
50	1.5	Scallops, baked or broiled
50	1.2	Scallops, steamed or boiled
95	10.0	Scallops, floured or breaded, fried

GI	GL	Food Name
95	12.4	Scallops, battered, fried
50	0.6	Shrimp, cooked
50	0.6	Shrimp, baked or broiled
50	0.6	Shrimp, steamed or boiled
95	11.2	Shrimp, floured, breaded, or battered, fried
50	0.0	Shrimp, canned
50	1.2	Snails, cooked

Meat, Poultry, Fish with Nonmeat Items

GI	GL	Food Name
37	1.4	Beef with tomato-based sauce (mixture)
38	3.2	Spaghetti sauce with beef or meat other than lamb or mutton, homemade-style
34	2.9	Chili con carne
34	2.9	Chili con carne with beans
37	2.1	Chili con carne without beans
34	2.7	Chili con carne, with cheese
34	2.7	Chili con carne with beans and cheese
42	3.7	Beef sloppy joe (no bun)
71	2.1	Beef with gravy (mixture)
64	3.8	Salisbury steak with gravy (mixture)
38	1.1	Beef with barbecue sauce (mixture)
50	3.5	Sausage gravy
34	2.9	Chili con carne with beans, made with pork
38	3.2	Spaghetti sauce with lamb or mutton, homemade-style
34	3.0	Chili con carne with venison/deer and beans

GI	GL	Food Name
61	3.2	Chicken or turkey cacciatore
38	3.2	Spaghetti sauce with poultry, home-made style
34	2.7	Chili con carne with chicken or turkey and beans
50	1.3	Turkey with gravy (mixture)
57	3.5	Chicken or turkey teriyaki (chicken or turkey with soy-based sauce)
38	0.9	Chicken or turkey with barbecue sauce (mixture), skin eaten
38	0.9	Chicken or turkey with barbecue sauce (mixture), skin not eaten
53	6.0	Sweet and sour chicken or turkey
82	4.0	Chicken or turkey cordon bleu
79	6.7	Chicken or turkey parmigiana
27	1.1	Clam sauce, white
0	0.0	Sardines with tomato-based sauce (mixture)
0	0.0	Sardines with mustard sauce (mixture)
38	2.9	Spaghetti sauce with combination of meats, homemade-style
70	6.8	Beef stew with potatoes, tomato-based sauce (mixture)
40	3.8	Beef and noodles with tomato-based sauce (mixture)
41	5.6	Chili con carne with beans and macaroni
46	4.0	Beef stroganoff with noodles
55	9.9	Chili con carne with beans and rice
61	4.0	Meat loaf made with beef
56	3.8	Meat loaf made with beef, with tomato-based sauce

MEAT, POULTRY, FISH and MIXTURES

GI	GL	Food Name
40	6.2	Chicken or turkey and noodles, no sauce (mixture)
46	6.6	Chicken or turkey and noodles with cream or white sauce (mixture)
91	8.1	Chicken or turkey with dumplings (mixture)
95	12.2	Chicken or turkey cake, patty, or croquette
60	4.5	Meat loaf made with chicken or turkey
79	9.0	Tuna cake or patty
59	9.0	Tuna noodle casserole with cream or white sauce
52	7.4	Tuna noodle casserole with (mushroom) soup
52	6.9	Tuna and rice with (mushroom) soup (mixture)
50	6.4	Liver dumpling
63	4.9	Beef stew with potatoes and vegetables (including carrots, broccoli, and/or dark-green leafy), tomato-based sauce
64	5.6	Beef stew with potatoes and vegetables (including carrots, broccoli, and/or dark-green leafy), gravy
35	3.2	Beef, noodles, and vegetables (excluding carrots, broccoli, and dark-green leafy), (mushroom) soup
47	5.9	Beef, rice, and vegetables (including carrots, broccoli, and/or dark-green leafy), (mushroom) soup (mixture)
49	5.8	Beef, rice, and vegetables (excluding carrots, broccoli, and dark-green leafy), (mushroom) soup (mixture)
45	7.8	Beef pot pie
85	14.0	Chicken or turkey pot pie
51	8.1	Tuna noodle casserole with vegetables, cream or white sauce

GI	GL	Food Name
52	7.6	Tuna noodle casserole with vegetables and (mushroom) soup
50	1.9	Swiss steak
38	2.4	Beef with vegetables (including carrots, broccoli, and/or dark-green leafy (no potatoes)), (mushroom) soup (mixture)
38	1.8	Beef with vegetables (excluding carrots, broccoli, and dark-green leafy (no potatoes)), (mushroom) soup (mixture)
49	2.2	Beef and vegetables (including carrots, broccoli, and/or dark-green leafy (no potatoes)), soy-based sauce (mixture)
46	1.1	Pepper steak
50	1.9	Seasoned shredded soup meat (Ropa vieja, sopa de carne ripiada)
43	2.9	Chicken or turkey and vegetables (including carrots, broccoli, and/or dark-green leafy (no potatoes)), no sauce (mixture)
55	3.2	Chicken or turkey and vegetables (including carrots, broccoli, and/or dark-green leafy (no potatoes)), soy-based sauce (mixture)
41	0.6	Chicken or turkey salad
32	0.8	Chicken or turkey garden salad (chicken and/or turkey, tomato and/or carrots, other vegetables), no dressing
0	0.0	Chicken or turkey fricassee, no sauce, no potatoes, Puerto Rican style
39	2.7	Tuna salad
40	2.5	Tuna salad with egg

MEAT, POULTRY, FISH and MIXTURES

GI	GL	Food Name
64	6.3	Tuna casserole with vegetables and (mushroom) soup, no noodles
50	3.5	Liver, beef or calves, and onions
70	13.4	Roast beef sandwich
69	11.7	Roast beef sandwich with cheese
67	16.3	Chicken patty sandwich, with lettuce and spread
69	15.6	Chicken fillet, (broiled), sandwich, on whole wheat roll, with lettuce, tomato and spread
59	10.4	Chicken fillet, broiled, sandwich with cheese, on bun, with lettuce, tomato and spread

Frozen Meals, Soups and Gravies

GI	GL	Food Name
50	0.0	Beef, broth, bouillon, or consomme
38	1.3	Oxtail soup
38	0.6	Beef broth, with tomato, home recipe
51	4.4	Chili beef soup
51	3.2	Chili beef soup, chunky style
38	1.4	Meatball soup, Mexican style (Sopa de Albondigas)
42	2.6	Beef noodle soup, Puerto Rican style (Sopa de carne y fideos)
53	3.7	Beef and rice noodle soup, Oriental style (Vietnamese Pho Bo)
38	1.5	Pepperpot (tripe) soup
44	3.6	Beef vegetable soup with potato, stew type
40	3.8	Beef vegetable soup with noodles, stew type, chunky
51	4.9	Beef vegetable soup with rice, stew type, chunky style
38	2.0	Beef vegetable soup, Mexican style (Sopa / caldo de Res)

GI	GL	Food Name
40	2.5	Meat and corn hominy soup, Mexican style (Pozole)
42	3.8	Beef stroganoff soup, chunky style
51	1.6	Pork and rice soup, stew type, chunky style
40	1.3	Pork vegetable soup with noodles, stew type, chunky
51	4.0	Ham, rice, and potato soup, Puerto Rican style
38	2.6	Pork, vegetable soup with potatoes, stew type
38	0.2	Pork with vegetable (excluding carrots, broccoli and/or dark-green leafy) soup, Oriental Style
32	1.2	Scotch broth (lamb, vegetables, and barley)
50	0.2	Chicken, broth, bouillon, or consomme
38	1.4	Chicken broth, with tomato, home recipe
50	0.2	Chicken broth, canned, less or reduced sodium
0	0.0	Chicken broth, canned, low sodium
64	5.3	Chicken rice soup, Puerto Rican style (Sopa de pollo con arroz)
57	4.8	Chicken soup with noodles and potatoes, Puerto Rican style
38	1.3	Chicken gumbo soup
40	2.8	Chicken noodle soup, chunky style
42	1.6	Chicken soup
38	0.7	Chicken soup with vegetables (broccoli, carrots, celery, potatoes and onions), Oriental style
38	2.6	Chicken or turkey vegetable soup, stew type
51	2.8	Chicken vegetable soup with rice, stew type, chunky style

MEAT, POULTRY, FISH and MIXTURES

GI	GL	Food Name
40	3.2	Chicken vegetable soup with noodles, stew type, chunky style
38	2.0	Chicken or turkey vegetable soup, home recipe
51	5.3	Chicken vegetable soup with rice, Mexican style (Sopa / Caldo de Pollo)
44	2.3	Chicken vegetable soup with potato and cheese, chunky style
27	1.9	Chicken or turkey soup, cream of, canned, reduced sodium, made with milk
27	1.3	Chicken or turkey soup, cream of, canned, reduced sodium, made with water
27	1.3	Chicken or turkey soup, cream of
27	1.6	Chicken or turkey soup, cream of, prepared with milk
27	1.0	Chicken or turkey soup, cream of, prepared with water
27	1.9	Chicken or turkey soup, cream of, canned, undiluted
27	1.7	Chicken and mushroom soup, cream of, prepared with milk
0	0.0	Fish stock, home recipe
27	1.3	Fish chowder
38	1.9	Crab soup, tomato-base
30	2.3	Clam chowder, NS as to Manhattan or New England style
38	2.4	Clam chowder, Manhattan
27	1.8	Clam chowder, New England, NS as to prepared with water or milk
27	1.8	Clam chowder, New England, prepared with milk
27	1.4	Clam chowder, New England, prepared with water

GI	GL	Food Name
27	2.2	Clam chowder, New England, canned, reduced sodium, ready-to-serve
27	1.3	Crab soup, cream of, prepared with milk
27	0.7	Salmon soup, cream style
27	1.3	Shrimp soup, cream of, prepared with milk
50	2.7	Gravy, poultry
50	2.2	Gravy, meat or poultry, with wine
50	3.5	Gravy, meat, with fruit
50	3.1	Gravy, poultry, low sodium
50	2.4	Gravy, beef or meat
50	2.4	Gravy, giblet
50	2.7	Gravy, mushroom
50	0.0	Gravy, redeye
50	2.9	Gravy or sauce, poultry-based from Puerto Rican-style chicken fricasse
50	4.6	Gravy or sauce, Chinese (soy sauce, stock or bouillon, cornstarch)

EGGS

GI	GL	Food Name
50	0.4	Egg, whole, raw
50	0.6	Egg, whole, cooked
50	0.6	Egg, whole, boiled
50	0.4	Egg, whole, poached

EGGS

GI	GL	Food Name
50	0.5	Egg, whole, fried
50	0.4	Egg, whole, fried without fat
50	0.5	Egg, whole, baked
50	0.4	Egg, whole, baked, fat not added in cooking
50	0.5	Egg, whole, baked, fat added in cooking
50	0.6	Egg, whole, pickled
50	0.4	Egg, white only, raw
50	0.4	Egg, white only, cooked
50	1.8	Egg, yolk only, raw
50	1.8	Egg, yolk only, cooked
50	0.7	Duck egg, cooked
50	0.7	Goose egg, cooked
50	0.2	Quail egg, canned
50	0.7	Egg, deviled
50	1.0	Egg salad
50	0.6	Egg, scrambled, made from dry eggs
50	0.9	Egg omelet or scrambled egg
50	1.0	Egg omelet or scrambled egg, fat not added in cooking
50	1.0	Egg omelet or scrambled egg, fat added in cooking
50	1.5	Egg omelet or scrambled egg, with cheese
50	0.9	Egg omelet or scrambled egg, with fish
50	0.7	Egg omelet or scrambled egg, with ham or bacon
50	1.4	Egg omelet or scrambled egg, with dark-green vegetables

GI	GL	Food Name
50	1.5	Egg omelet or scrambled egg, with vegetables other than dark-green vegetables
50	1.3	Egg omelet or scrambled egg, with peppers, onion, and ham
50	1.4	Egg omelet or scrambled egg, with mushrooms
50	1.3	Egg omelet or scrambled egg, with cheese and ham or bacon
50	1.5	Egg omelet or scrambled egg, with cheese, ham or bacon, and tomatoes
50	4.6	Egg omelet or scrambled egg, with potatoes and/or onions (Tortilla Espanola, traditional style Spanish
50	1.3	Egg omelet or scrambled egg, with beef
50	1.0	Egg omelet or scrambled egg, with sausage and mushrooms
50	1.3	Egg omelet or scrambled egg, with sausage and cheese
50	0.8	Egg omelet or scrambled egg, with sausage
50	1.4	Egg omelet or scrambled egg, with hot dogs
50	2.0	Egg omelet or scrambled egg, with onions, peppers, tomatoes, and mushrooms
50	1.8	Egg omelet or scrambled egg, with chili, cheese, tomatoes, and beans
50	1.0	Egg omelet or scrambled egg, with chorizo
50	0.7	Egg omelet or scrambled egg with chicken
50	4.3	Huevos rancheros
50	4.8	Shrimp-egg patty (Torta de Cameron seco)
50	0.4	Egg substitute

GI	GL	Food Name
50	2.3	Scrambled egg, made from powdered mixture
50	2.0	Scrambled egg, made from cholesterol-free frozen mixture
50	2.4	Scrambled egg, made from cholesterol-free frozen mixture with cheese
50	1.3	Scrambled egg, made from cholesterol-free frozen mixture with vegetables
50	3.3	Scrambled egg, made from frozen mixture
50	1.0	Scrambled egg, made from packaged liquid mixture

LEGUMES, NUTS and SEEDS

Legumes

GI	GL	Food Name
29	6.1	Beans, dry, cooked
29	6.1	Beans, dry, cooked, fat added in cooking
29	6.6	Beans, dry, cooked, fat not added in cooking
13	3.0	White beans, dry, cooked
13	3.0	White beans, dry, cooked, fat added in cooking
13	3.2	White beans, dry, cooked, fat not added in cooking
20	3.9	Black, brown, or Bayo beans, dry, cooked, fat added in cooking
20	4.2	Black, brown, or Bayo beans, dry, cooked, fat not added in cooking
31	5.9	Lima beans, dry, cooked
31	5.9	Lima beans, dry, cooked, fat added in cooking
31	6.4	Lima beans, dry, cooked, fat not added in cooking
39	7.4	Pinto, calico, or red Mexican beans, dry, cooked, fat added in cooking

GI	GL	Food Name
39	8.1	Pinto, calico, or red Mexican beans, dry, cooked, fat not added in cooking
28	5.8	Red kidney beans, dry, cooked
28	5.8	Red kidney beans, dry, cooked, fat added in cooking
28	6.3	Red kidney beans, dry, cooked, fat not added in cooking
16	1.6	Soybeans, cooked, fat not added in cooking
37	7.4	Mung beans, fat not added in cooking
37	6.8	Mung beans, fat added in cooking
48	9.8	Baked beans
48	10.1	Baked beans, vegetarian
48	8.1	Chili beans, barbecue beans, ranch style beans or Mexican- style beans
48	10.6	Boston baked beans
42	7.9	Refried beans
48	9.3	Beans, dry, cooked with ground beef
48	9.0	Pork and beans
48	11.5	Beans, dry, cooked with pork
28	5.5	Stewed dry red beans, Puerto Rican style (Habichuelas coloradas guisadas)
31	1.2	Stewed dry lima beans, Puerto Rican style
48	9.9	Baked beans, low sodium
42	8.0	Cowpeas, dry, cooked
42	8.0	Cowpeas, dry, cooked, fat added in cooking
42	8.7	Cowpeas, dry, cooked, fat not added in cooking
28	7.7	Chickpeas, dry, cooked

LEGUMES, NUTS and SEEDS

GI	GL	Food Name
28	7.7	Chickpeas, dry, cooked, fat added in cooking
28	8.4	Chickpeas, dry, cooked, fat not added in cooking
32	6.7	Green or yellow split peas, dry, cooked, fat not added in cooking
32	6.3	Green or yellow split peas, dry, cooked, fat added in cooking
32	6.3	Green or yellow split peas, dry, cooked
42	5.8	Cowpeas, dry, cooked with pork
28	5.3	Lentils, dry, cooked
28	5.3	Lentils, dry, cooked, fat added in cooking
28	5.7	Lentils, dry, cooked, fat not added in cooking
28	2.2	Chickpeas stewed with pig's feet, Puerto Rican style (Garbanzos guisados con patitos de cerdo)
16	0.3	Soybean curd
16	1.7	Soybean curd, deep fried
16	1.5	Soybean curd, breaded, fried
16	5.6	Soybean meal
40	5.8	Meal replacement or supplement, soy- and milk-base, powder, reconstituted with water
56	34.9	High protein bar, candy-like, soy and milk base
45	6.8	Meal replacement or supplement, liquid, soy-base, high protein
50	8.2	Ensure with fiber, liquid
40	8.0	Ensure Plus liquid nutrition
40	5.6	Meal replacement or supplement, liquid, soy-based

GI	GL	Food Name
115	28.4	Tofu, frozen dessert, chocolate
64	4.9	Bean soup
64	5.8	Bean with bacon or pork soup
64	5.1	Black bean soup
60	3.9	Lima bean soup
44	2.3	Soybean soup, made with milk
38	3.1	Bean soup, with macaroni and meat
29	0.9	Soybean soup, miso broth
38	3.5	Bean soup, with macaroni
64	7.6	Bean and ham soup, chunky style
64	5.8	Bean soup, mixed beans
64	6.8	Bean soup, home recipe
42	3.9	Bean and rice soup
64	4.6	Bean and ham soup, home recipe
66	7.4	Chunky pea and ham soup
64	9.0	Garbanzo or chickpea soup
60	6.7	Split pea and ham soup
66	5.5	Pea soup, instant type
60	6.4	Split pea soup
60	7.1	Split pea soup, canned, reduced sodium, prepared with water or ready-to-serve
60	6.8	Split pea and ham soup, canned, reduced sodium, prepared with water or ready-to-serve
44	4.7	Lentil soup

GI	GL	Food Name
16	2.1	Soyburger, meatless, no bun
39	2.7	Vegetarian stew

Nuts and Seeds

GI	GL	Food Name
22	6.6	Cashew nuts
22	6.6	Cashew nuts, roasted (assume salted)
22	6.6	Cashew nuts, roasted, without salt
22	7.2	Cashew nuts, dry roasted
18	3.9	Mixed nuts
18	3.9	Mixed nuts, roasted, with peanuts
22	4.9	Mixed nuts, roasted, without peanuts
18	4.6	Mixed nuts, dry roasted
18	5.3	Mixed nuts, honey-roasted, with peanuts
18	2.5	Mixed nuts, in shell
14	2.1	Peanuts
14	3.0	Peanuts, boiled
14	2.1	Peanuts, roasted, salted
14	2.6	Peanuts, roasted, without salt
14	3.0	Peanuts, dry roasted, salted
14	3.0	Peanuts, dry roasted, without salt
14	3.3	Peanuts, honey-roasted
20	2.8	Pecans
20	2.7	Walnuts
22	6.1	Cashew butter
14	2.7	Peanut butter

GI	GL	Food Name
14	2.7	Peanut butter, low sodium
14	3.1	Peanut butter, reduced sodium
14	5.0	Peanut butter, reduced fat
20	3.8	Sunflower seeds, hulled, unroasted

GRAIN PRODUCTS

Yeast Breads, Rolls

GI	GL	Food Name
70	35.4	Bread
73	39.7	Bread, toasted
70	34.7	Bread
73	40.0	Bread, toasted
70	34.6	Roll
73	39.7	Roll, toasted
70	37.4	Roll
73	38.5	Roll, hard
70	35.4	Bread, white
73	39.7	Bread, white, toasted
70	33.9	Bread, white with whole wheat swirl
70	37.1	Bread, white with whole wheat swirl, toasted
95	49.4	Bread, Cuban
95	54.3	Bread, Cuban, toasted
70	36.4	Bread, Native, Puerto Rican style (Pan Criollo)
73	41.7	Bread, Native, Puerto Rican style, toasted (Pan Criollo)
95	49.3	Bread, French or Vienna
95	53.6	Bread, French or Vienna, toasted

GRAIN PRODUCTS

GI	GL	Food Name
70	35.0	Bread, Italian, Grecian, Armenian
73	40.1	Bread, Italian, Grecian, Armenian, toasted
57	31.7	Bread, pita
57	34.9	Bread, pita, toasted
70	35.4	Bread, cinnamon
73	39.7	Bread, cinnamon, toasted
95	47.5	Bread, lowfat, 98% fat free
95	52.2	Bread, lowfat, 98% fat free, toasted
95	43.3	Bread, garlic
95	47.6	Bread, garlic, toasted
68	30.1	Bread, reduced calorie and/or high fiber, white
68	33.1	Bread, reduced calorie and/or high fiber, white, toasted
68	28.9	Bread, reduced calorie and/or high fiber, Italian
68	31.7	Bread, reduced calorie and/or high fiber, Italian, toasted
68	30.3	Bread, reduced calorie and/or high fiber, white, with fruit and/or nuts
68	33.3	Bread, reduced calorie and/or high fiber, white, with fruit and/or nuts, toasted
68	34.4	Bread, white, special formula, added fiber
63	32.9	Bread, raisin
63	35.8	Bread, raisin, toasted
70	34.7	Bread, white, low sodium or no salt
73	39.7	Bread, white, low sodium or no salt, toasted
54	28.0	Bread, sour dough

GI	GL	Food Name
54	30.5	Bread, sour dough, toasted
66	29.6	Bread, dough, fried
70	34.6	Roll, white, soft
70	38.0	Roll, white, soft, toasted
70	37.4	Roll, white, soft
68	28.6	Roll, white, soft, reduced calorie and/or high fiber
68	31.5	Roll, white, soft, reduced calorie and/or high fiber,
73	38.5	Roll, white, hard
73	42.3	Roll, white, hard, toasted
95	47.7	Roll, French or Vienna
95	54.2	Roll, French or Vienna, toasted
73	36.7	Roll, garlic
73	36.1	Roll, hoagie, submarine
73	39.7	Roll, hoagie, submarine, toasted
73	37.7	Roll, Mexican, bolillo
54	28.0	Roll, sour dough
58	29.5	Roll, sweet
58	32.4	Roll, sweet, toasted
58	29.5	Roll, sweet, cinnamon bun, no frosting
58	32.8	Roll, sweet, cinnamon bun, frosted
58	30.6	Roll, sweet, with fruit, no frosting
58	34.2	Roll, sweet, with fruit, frosted
58	29.6	Roll, sweet, with fruit, frosted, diet
58	31.5	Roll, sweet, with nuts, frosted

GRAIN PRODUCTS

GI	GL	Food Name
58	34.2	Roll, sweet, with fruit, frosted, fat free
58	32.8	Roll, sweet, with fruit and nuts, frosted
58	28.3	Roll, sweet, with nuts, no frosting
59	33.1	Roll, sweet, no topping, Mexican (Pan Dulce)
59	36.1	Roll, sweet, crumb topping, Mexican (Pan Dulce)
59	33.3	Roll, sweet, sugar topping, Mexican (Pan Dulce)
58	29.5	Coffee cake, yeast type
58	32.8	Coffee cake, yeast type
58	36.0	Coffee cake, yeast type, fat free, cholesterol free, with fruit
67	30.7	Croissant
67	31.5	Croissant, cheese
67	29.6	Croissant, chocolate
67	29.3	Croissant, fruit
67	30.2	Croissant, nut
67	31.1	Brioche
72	36.4	Bagel
72	41.1	Bagel, toasted
72	39.7	Bagel, with raisins
72	42.7	Bagel, with raisins, toasted
72	39.3	Bagel, with fruit other than raisins
72	41.4	Bagel, with fruit other than raisins, toasted
74	16.1	Bread stuffing
74	15.1	Bread stuffing made with egg

GI	GL	Food Name
70	47.9	Bread sticks, hard
70	40.4	Bread stick, soft
70	47.9	Bread stick
70	35.9	Bread stick, soft, prepared with garlic and parmesan cheese
70	50.1	Bread stick, hard, low sodium
77	34.0	Muffin, English
77	40.5	Muffin, English, toasted
77	37.0	Muffin, English, with raisins
77	42.4	Muffin, English, with raisins, toasted
77	42.2	Muffin, English, with fruit other than raisins, toasted
70	53.6	Melba toast
71	32.7	Bread, whole wheat, 100%
71	36.7	Bread, whole wheat, 100%, toasted
71	35.1	Bread, whole wheat, 100%
71	38.6	Bread, whole wheat, 100%, toasted
71	35.4	Bread, whole wheat, 100%, with raisins
71	39.0	Bread, whole wheat, 100%, with raisins, toasted
71	39.1	Bread, pita, whole wheat, 100%
71	42.9	Bread, pita, whole wheat, 100%, toasted
71	28.7	Muffin, English, whole wheat, 100%
71	31.3	Muffin, English, whole wheat, 100%, toasted
71	36.8	Muffin, English, whole wheat, 100%, with raisins
71	41.2	Muffin, English, whole wheat, 100%, with raisins, toasted

GRAIN PRODUCTS

GI	GL	Food Name
53	27.2	Bread, sprouted wheat, toasted
71	40.0	Bagel, whole wheat, 100%
71	42.9	Bagel, whole wheat, 100%, toasted
71	38.1	Bagel, whole wheat, 100%, with raisins
71	41.0	Bagel, whole wheat, 100%, with raisins, toasted
71	36.3	Roll, whole wheat, 100%
71	39.9	Roll, whole wheat, 100%, toasted
71	33.2	Roll, whole wheat, 100%
71	36.1	Roll, whole wheat, 100%, toasted
71	33.5	Bread, whole wheat
71	36.4	Bread, whole wheat, toasted
71	36.5	Bread, whole wheat
71	40.0	Bread, whole wheat, toasted
71	33.2	Bread, puri or poori (Indian puffed bread), whole wheat, fried
71	36.1	Bread, whole wheat, with raisins
71	38.7	Bread, whole wheat, with raisins, toasted
71	33.5	Bread, wheat or cracked wheat
71	36.4	Bread, wheat or cracked wheat, toasted
53	27.1	Bread, wheat or cracked wheat
53	30.1	Bread, wheat or cracked wheat, toasted
53	27.0	Bread, wheat or cracked wheat, with raisins
53	28.9	Bread, wheat or cracked wheat, with raisins, toasted

GI	GL	Food Name
71	31.0	Bread, wheat or cracked wheat, reduced calorie and/or high fiber
71	34.0	Bread, wheat or cracked wheat, reduced calorie and/or high fiber, toasted
71	37.1	Bread, French or Vienna, whole wheat
71	41.2	Bread, French or Vienna, whole wheat, toasted
71	39.6	Bread, pita, whole wheat
71	44.0	Bread, pita, whole wheat, toasted
53	29.6	Bread, pita, wheat or cracked wheat
53	32.9	Bread, pita, wheat or cracked wheat, toasted
71	41.5	Bagel, wheat
71	44.4	Bagel, wheat, toasted
71	41.5	Bagel, whole wheat
71	44.4	Bagel, whole wheat, toasted
71	41.2	Bagel, wheat, with raisins
71	43.9	Bagel, wheat, with raisins, toasted
71	42.0	Bagel, wheat, with fruit and nuts
71	44.2	Bagel, wheat, with fruit and nuts, toasted
71	40.5	Bagel, wheat bran
71	43.4	Bagel, wheat bran, toasted
71	33.9	Bread, wheat bran
71	37.3	Bread, wheat bran, toasted
71	30.5	Muffin, English, wheat bran
71	35.0	Muffin, English, wheat bran, toasted

GRAIN PRODUCTS

GI	GL	Food Name
71	31.8	Muffin, English, wheat or cracked wheat
71	34.6	Muffin, English, wheat or cracked wheat, toasted
71	31.8	Muffin, English, whole wheat
71	34.6	Muffin, English, whole wheat, toasted
71	40.2	Muffin, English, wheat or cracked wheat, with raisins, toasted
71	40.2	Muffin, English, whole wheat, with raisins, toasted
83	56.8	Bread stick, hard, whole wheat
71	32.7	Roll, wheat or cracked wheat
71	35.9	Roll, wheat or cracked wheat, toasted
71	34.1	Roll, wheat or cracked wheat
71	37.4	Roll, wheat or cracked wheat, toasted
71	32.7	Roll, whole wheat
71	35.9	Roll, whole wheat, toasted
71	34.1	Roll, whole wheat
71	37.4	Roll, whole wheat, toasted
58	28.0	Bread, rye
58	30.8	Bread, rye, toasted
50	24.0	Bread, marble rye and pumpernickel
50	26.3	Bread, marble rye and pumpernickel, toasted
68	27.5	Bread, rye, reduced calorie and/or high fiber
68	30.3	Bread, rye, reduced calorie and/or high fiber, toasted
50	23.8	Bread, pumpernickel
50	26.1	Bread, pumpernickel, toasted

GI	GL	Food Name
50	29.3	Bagel, pumpernickel
50	31.4	Bagel, pumpernickel, toasted
76	36.1	Bread, black
76	39.7	Bread, black, toasted
58	30.8	Roll, rye
50	26.4	Roll, pumpernickel
50	29.0	Roll, pumpernickel, toasted
55	26.7	Bread, oatmeal
55	29.0	Bread, oatmeal, toasted
31	13.7	Bread, oat bran
31	13.5	Bread, oat bran, toasted
31	12.8	Bread, oat bran, reduced calorie and/or high fiber
31	15.3	Bread, oat bran, reduced calorie and/or high fiber,
47	25.1	Bagel, oat bran
47	26.4	Bagel, oat bran, toasted
47	20.3	Muffin, English, oat bran
47	26.1	Muffin, English, oat bran, toasted
43	21.7	Bread, multigrain, toasted
43	20.0	Bread, multigrain
43	21.6	Bread, multigrain, with raisins
43	23.8	Bread, multigrain, with raisins, toasted
43	22.5	Bread, multigrain, reduced calorie and/or high fiber
43	24.8	Bread, multigrain, reduced calorie and/or high fiber, toasted

GRAIN PRODUCTS

GI	GL	Food Name
43	19.2	Roll, multigrain
43	21.1	Roll, multigrain, toasted
43	22.6	Bagel, multigrain
43	23.7	Bagel, multigrain, toasted
43	23.9	Bagel, multigrain, with raisins
43	25.1	Bagel, multigrain, with raisins, toasted
43	19.9	Muffin, English, multigrain
43	21.6	Muffin, English, multigrain, toasted
67	36.6	Bread, barley
57	25.9	Bread, sunflower meal
67	31.5	Bread, rice, toasted
72	21.2	Injera (American-style Ethiopian bread)

Quick Breads

GI	GL	Food Name
92	43.1	Biscuit, baking powder or buttermilk type
66	30.5	Biscuit dough, fried
69	19.5	Crumpet
69	22.0	Crumpet, toasted
92	51.0	Biscuit, baking powder or buttermilk type, made from refrigerated dough, lowfat
92	43.7	Biscuit, baking powder or buttermilk type, made from refrigerated dough
92	41.0	Biscuit, baking powder or buttermilk type
92	41.8	Scone

GI	GL	Food Name
92	39.3	Scone, whole wheat
92	46.1	Scone, with fruit
76	26.3	Cornbread, prepared from mix
76	31.9	Cornbread
76	16.5	Cornbread stuffing
76	38.4	Cornbread muffin, stick, round
76	40.5	Cornbread muffin, stick, round, toasted
76	34.2	Cornbread muffin, stick, round
76	31.0	Corn flour patty or tart, fried
76	29.0	Corn pone, baked
76	34.7	Hush puppy
76	13.7	Spoonbread
41	19.7	Tortilla
52	23.2	Tortilla, corn
30	15.4	Tortilla, flour (wheat)
30	16.7	Tortilla, whole wheat
61	30.3	Muffin
59	28.3	Muffin, fruit and/or nuts
59	34.8	Muffin, fruit, fat free, cholesterol free
53	24.2	Muffin, chocolate chip
53	22.9	Muffin, chocolate
60	25.5	Muffin, whole wheat
60	26.2	Muffin, wheat
60	25.8	Muffin, buckwheat

GRAIN PRODUCTS

GI	GL	Food Name
60	31.3	Muffin, wheat bran
60	31.9	Muffin, bran with fruit, lowfat
60	32.0	Muffin, bran with fruit, no fat, no cholesterol
69	26.6	Muffin, oatmeal
60	29.0	Muffin, oat bran
60	28.9	Muffin, oat bran with fruit and/or nuts
44	19.3	Muffin, plain
62	36.5	Muffin, pumpkin
58	27.3	Muffin, zucchini
62	27.6	Muffin, carrot
65	27.4	Muffin, multigrain, with nuts
58	25.8	Bread, nut
58	32.6	Bread, pumpkin
58	31.6	Bread, fruit, without nuts
58	30.5	Bread, fruit and nut
58	24.9	Bread, whole wheat, with nuts
58	27.3	Bread, zucchini

Cakes, Cookies, Pies, Pastries

GI	GL	Food Name
42	23.3	Cake, with or without icing
67	38.3	Cake, angel food, without icing
67	42.4	Cake, angel food, with icing
67	25.1	Cake, angel food, with fruit and icing or filling
67	37.9	Cake, angel food, chocolate, without icing
44	28.3	Cake, applesauce

GI	GL	Food Name
44	26.0	Cake, applesauce, without icing
44	28.3	Cake, applesauce, with icing
47	26.6	Cake, banana
47	24.6	Cake, banana, without icing
47	26.6	Cake, banana, with icing
38	14.4	Cake, black forest (chocolate-cherry)
42	21.1	Cake, butter, without icing
42	25.3	Cake, butter, with icing
62	32.8	Cake, carrot
62	30.4	Cake, carrot, without icing
62	32.8	Cake, carrot, with icing
42	26.5	Cake, coconut, with icing
50	14.6	Cheesecake
50	15.1	Cheesecake, diet
50	16.5	Cheesecake with fruit
50	15.0	Cheesecake, diet, with fruit
50	19.2	Cheesecake, chocolate
50	15.9	Cheesecake, chocolate, reduced fat
38	23.4	Cake, chocolate, devil's food, or fudge
38	20.0	Cake, chocolate, devil's food, or fudge, standard-type mix (eggs and water added to dry mix), without icing or
38	19.5	Cake, chocolate, devil's food, or fudge, without icing or filling

GRAIN PRODUCTS

GI	GL	Food Name
38	24.1	Cake, chocolate, devil's food, or fudge, standard-type mix (eggs and water added to dry mix), with icing, coating, or filling
38	23.4	Cake, chocolate, devil's food, or fudge, with icing, coating, or filling
38	18.8	Cake, German chocolate, with icing and filling
38	21.3	Cake, chocolate, with icing, diet
38	23.4	Cake, chocolate, devil's food, or fudge, pudding-type mix, made by "Lite" recipe (eggs and water added to dry mix, no oil added to dry mix), with icing, coating, or filling
38	20.9	Cake, chocolate, devil's food, or fudge, pudding type mix, made by "cholesterol free" recipe (water, oil and egg whites added to dry mix), with "light" icing, coating or filling
38	21.5	Cake, chocolate, devil's food, or fudge, pudding-type mix (oil, eggs, and water added to dry mix)
38	16.8	Cake, chocolate, devil's food, or fudge, pudding-type mix (oil, eggs, and water added to dry mix), without icing or filling
38	21.5	Cake, chocolate, devil's food, or fudge, pudding-type mix (oil, eggs, and water added to dry mix), with icing, coating, or filling
42	28.4	Cake, cupcake
42	28.5	Cake, cupcake, with icing
38	24.2	Cake, cupcake, chocolate
38	20.0	Cake, cupcake, chocolate, without icing or filling
38	22.9	Cake, cupcake, chocolate, with icing or filling
58	36.1	Cake, cupcake, not chocolate

GI	GL	Food Name
58	31.3	Cake, cupcake, not chocolate, without icing or filling
58	36.7	Cake, cupcake, not chocolate, with icing or filling
73	48.0	Cake, cupcake, not chocolate, with icing or filling, lowfat, cholesterol free
58	32.4	Cake, cupcake, not chocolate, with fruit and cream filling
38	24.6	Cake, cupcake, chocolate, with or without icing, fruit filling or cream filling, lowfat, cholesterol free
38	17.9	Cake, Dobos Torte (non-chocolate layer cake with chocolate filling and icing)
58	35.7	Cake, fruit cake, light or dark, holiday type cake
58	27.1	Cake, plum pudding
58	29.3	Cake, gingerbread, without icing
50	19.9	Cake, ice cream and cake roll, chocolate
52	19.4	Cake, ice cream and cake roll, not chocolate
50	24.2	Cake, frozen yogurt and cake layer, not chocolate, with icing
50	22.7	Cake, frozen yogurt and cake layer, chocolate, with icing
42	23.2	Cake, lemon
42	21.1	Cake, lemon, without icing
42	27.2	Cake, lemon, with icing
42	27.1	Cake, lemon, lowfat
42	23.5	Cake, lemon, lowfat, without icing
42	27.1	Cake, lemon, lowfat, with icing
40	24.6	Cake, marble
40	23.5	Cake, marble, without icing

GRAIN PRODUCTS

GI	GL	Food Name
40	24.6	Cake, marble, with icing
42	24.0	Cake, nut
42	18.6	Cake, nut, without icing
42	23.0	Cake, nut, with icing
42	19.9	Cake, poppyseed, without icing
54	29.3	Cake, pound, without icing
54	32.0	Cake, pound, with icing
54	29.0	Cake, pound, chocolate
54	32.4	Cake, pound, chocolate, fat free, cholesterol free
54	32.9	Cake, pound, fat free, cholesterol free
54	29.9	Cake, pound, reduced fat, cholesterol free
62	34.9	Cake, pumpkin
62	31.6	Cake, pumpkin, without icing
62	34.9	Cake, pumpkin, with icing
54	31.5	Cake, raisin-nut, without icing
42	23.5	Cake, spice
42	23.2	Cake, spice, without icing
42	23.5	Cake, spice, with icing
46	31.0	Cake, sponge
46	28.1	Cake, sponge, without icing
46	31.0	Cake, sponge, with icing
87	50.4	Cake, sponge, chocolate, with icing
44	22.3	Cake, upside down (all fruits)

GI	GL	Food Name
42	30.8	Cake, white, standard-type mix (egg whites and water added)
42	27.0	Cake, white
42	25.2	Cake, white, standard-type mix (egg whites and water added to mix), without icing
42	22.1	Cake, white, without icing
42	28.6	Cake, white, standard-type mix (egg whites and water added to mix), with icing
42	27.1	Cake, white, with icing
42	25.6	Cake, white, pudding-type mix (oil, egg whites, and water added to dry mix)
42	21.5	Cake, white, pudding-type mix (oil, egg whites, and water added to dry mix), without icing
42	25.6	Cake, white, pudding-type mix (oil, egg whites, and water added to dry mix), with icing
42	27.0	Cake, yellow, standard-type mix (eggs and water added to dry mix)
42	27.2	Cake, yellow
42	22.9	Cake, yellow, standard-type mix (eggs and water added to dry mix), without icing
42	24.2	Cake, yellow, without icing
42	27.0	Cake, yellow, standard-type mix (eggs and water added to dry mix), with icing
42	27.2	Cake, yellow, with icing
42	24.7	Cake, yellow, pudding-type mix (oil, eggs, and water added to dry mix)
42	20.2	Cake, yellow, pudding-type mix (oil, eggs, and water added to dry mix), without icing

GRAIN PRODUCTS

GI	GL	Food Name
42	24.7	Cake, yellow, pudding-type mix (oil, eggs, and water added to dry mix), with icing
58	32.2	Cake, zucchini, without icing
58	31.4	Cake, zucchini, with icing
64	34.8	Cookie, batter or dough, raw, not chocolate
57	39.0	Cookie
64	33.0	Cookie, almond
51	31.9	Cookie, brownie
51	31.9	Cookie, brownie, without icing
51	32.6	Cookie, brownie, with icing
51	28.4	Cookie, brownie, with cream cheese filling, without icing
51	30.3	Cookie, brownie, with peanut butter fudge icing
51	36.4	Cookie, brownie, diet
51	36.7	Cookie, brownie, lowfat, with icing
51	35.8	Cookie, brownie, lowfat, without icing
51	33.9	Cookie, brownie, fat free, cholesterol free, with icing
51	35.1	Cookie, brownie, fat free, without icing
53	30.3	Cookie, butterscotch, brownie
64	37.6	Cookie, butterscotch chip
49	31.4	Cookie, chocolate chip
49	31.9	Cookie, chocolate chip, with raisins
49	28.5	Cookie, chocolate chip
42	29.7	Cookie, chocolate chip, reduced fat
49	26.9	Cookie, rich, chocolate chip, with chocolate filling

GI	GL	Food Name
49	35.2	Cookie, chocolate chip sandwich
49	35.5	Cookie, chocolate fudge, with/without nuts
42	33.9	Cookie, chocolate, with chocolate filling or coating, fat free
49	35.1	Cookie, chocolate, chocolate sandwich or chocolate-coated or striped
42	34.9	Cookie, chocolate sandwich, reduced fat
49	32.4	Cookie, chocolate-covered, chocolate sandwich
49	33.4	Cookie, chocolate, sandwich, with extra filling
49	35.2	Cookie, chocolate and vanilla sandwich
74	52.3	Cookie, graham cracker sandwich with chocolate and marshmallow filling
51	36.2	Cookie, fruit-filled bar
51	39.2	Cookie, fruit-filled bar, fat free
51	36.2	Cookie, date bar
51	36.2	Cookie, fig bar
51	39.9	Cookie, fig bar, fat free
77	64.7	Cookie, fortune
65	51.4	Cookie, cone shell, ice cream type, wafer or cake
65	54.7	Cookie, cone shell, ice cream type, brown sugar
77	59.2	Cookie, gingersnaps
54	37.1	Cookie, oatmeal
54	37.1	Cookie, oatmeal, with raisins
54	34.4	Cookie, oatmeal, with fruit filling
54	42.4	Cookie, oatmeal, fat free, with raisins

GRAIN PRODUCTS

GI	GL	Food Name
54	41.9	Cookie, oatmeal, reduced fat, with raisins
54	37.1	Cookie, oatmeal sandwich, with creme filling
54	29.0	Cookie, oatmeal, with chocolate chips
64	37.7	Cookie, peanut butter
64	37.7	Cookie, peanut
64	41.3	Cookie, shortbread
64	46.2	Cookie, shortbread, reduced fat
57	36.3	Cookie, shortbread, with chocolate filling
55	36.1	Cookie, butter or sugar cookie
55	36.0	Cookie, butter or sugar cookie, with fruit and/or nuts
77	55.5	Cookie, vanilla sandwich
77	63.5	Cookie, vanilla sandwich, reduced fat
49	26.9	Cookie, rich, all chocolate, with chocolate filling or chocolate chips
49	33.7	Cookie, butter or sugar, with chocolate icing or filling
77	54.0	Cookie, vanilla waffle creme
55	51.1	Cookie, tea, Japanese
77	56.7	Cookie, vanilla wafer
77	60.7	Cookie, vanilla wafer, reduced fat
63	37.0	Cookie, vanilla with caramel, coconut, and chocolate coating
58	40.5	Cookie, dietetic, oatmeal with raisins
58	44.5	Cookie, dietetic, sugar or plain
59	20.1	Pie

GI	GL	Food Name
59	24.0	Pie, individual size or tart
59	20.1	Pie, apple, two crust
59	23.7	Pie, apple, individual size or tart
59	24.5	Pie, apple, fried pie
59	23.0	Pie, apple, one crust
59	26.4	Pie, apple, diet
59	23.1	Pie, apricot, two crust
59	24.1	Pie, apricot, fried pie
59	21.1	Pie, blackberry, two crust
59	21.8	Pie, blackberry, individual size or tart
59	23.5	Pie, berry, not blackberry, blueberry, boysenberry, huckleberry, raspberry, or strawberry; two crust
59	23.0	Pie, berry, not blackberry, blueberry, boysenberry, huckleberry, raspberry, or strawberry; one crust
59	24.1	Pie, berry, not blackberry, blueberry, boysenberry, huckleberry, raspberry, or strawberry, individual size or tart
59	20.6	Pie, blueberry, two crust
59	19.2	Pie, blueberry, one crust
59	23.1	Pie, blueberry, individual size or tart
59	23.5	Pie, cherry, two crust
59	21.7	Pie, cherry, one crust
59	19.1	Pie, cherry, individual size or tart
59	22.7	Pie, cherry, fried pie
59	33.9	Pie, lemon (not cream or meringue)

GRAIN PRODUCTS

GI	GL	Food Name
59	33.7	Pie, lemon (not cream or meringue), individual size or
59	21.5	Pie, lemon, fried pie
59	28.3	Pie, mince, two crust
59	24.7	Pie, mince, individual size or tart
59	19.4	Pie, peach, two crust
59	21.8	Pie, peach, one crust
59	22.3	Pie, peach, individual size or tart
59	22.7	Pie, peach, fried pie
59	22.0	Pie, pear, two crust
59	22.6	Pie, pear, individual size or tart
59	21.8	Pie, pineapple, two crust
59	22.2	Pie, pineapple, individual size or tart
59	24.1	Pie, plum, two crust
59	30.3	Pie, prune, one crust
59	21.8	Pie, raisin, two crust
59	23.9	Pie, raisin, individual size or tart
59	22.4	Pie, raspberry, one crust
59	22.7	Pie, raspberry, two crust
59	21.7	Pie, rhubarb, two crust
59	21.0	Pie, rhubarb, one crust
59	22.3	Pie, rhubarb, individual size or tart
59	20.4	Pie, strawberry, one crust
59	21.0	Pie, strawberry-rhubarb, two crust
59	21.4	Pie, strawberry, individual size or tart

GI	GL	Food Name
59	23.3	Pie, cherry, made with cream cheese and sour cream
59	19.4	Pie, banana cream
59	18.3	Pie, banana cream, individual size or tart
59	30.4	Pie, buttermilk
59	31.5	Pie, chess
59	20.6	Pie, chocolate cream
59	21.4	Pie, chocolate cream, individual size or tart
59	21.9	Pie, coconut cream
59	15.0	Pie, coconut cream, individual size or tart
59	12.3	Pie, custard
59	15.6	Pie, custard, individual size or tart
59	22.9	Pie, lemon cream
59	22.9	Pie, lemon cream, individual size or tart
59	19.9	Pie, peanut butter cream
59	17.6	Pie, pineapple cream
59	16.1	Pie, pumpkin
59	13.4	Pie, pumpkin, individual size or tart
59	13.6	Pie, raspberry cream
59	20.3	Pie, sour cream, raisin
59	15.2	Pie, squash
59	15.5	Pie, strawberry cream
59	17.0	Pie, strawberry cream, individual size or tart
59	12.3	Pie, sweetpotato
59	19.2	Pie, vanilla cream

GRAIN PRODUCTS

GI	GL	Food Name
59	27.8	Pie, lemon meringue
59	20.6	Pie, lemon meringue, individual size or tart
59	27.1	Pie, chocolate-marshmallow
59	33.7	Pie, pecan
59	31.4	Pie, pecan, individual size or tart
59	35.5	Pie, oatmeal
59	15.9	Pie, pudding, flavors other than chocolate
59	21.2	Pie, pudding, flavors other than chocolate, individual size or tart
59	23.3	Pie, pudding, chocolate, with chocolate coating, individual size
59	24.1	Pie, pudding, flavors other than chocolate, with chocolate coating, individual size
59	26.4	Pie, Toll house chocolate chip
46	16.8	Cobbler, apple
55	19.7	Cobbler, apricot
59	25.5	Cobbler, berry
55	19.6	Cobbler, cherry
55	20.2	Cobbler, peach
55	22.5	Cobbler, pear
59	21.7	Cobbler, pineapple
55	21.1	Cobbler, plum
55	25.8	Cobbler, rhubarb
49	15.1	Crisp, apple, apple dessert
59	19.2	Fritter, apple

GI	GL	Food Name
59	27.1	Crisp, cherry
59	21.4	Crisp, peach
59	25.4	Crisp, rhubarb
59	14.3	Cream puff, eclair, custard or cream filled
59	13.5	Cream puff, eclair, custard or cream filled, not iced
59	14.3	Cream puff, eclair, custard or cream filled, iced
59	24.7	Cream puff, eclair, custard or cream filled, iced, reduced fat
59	23.8	Air filled fritter or fried puff, without syrup, Puerto Rican style (Bunuelos de viento)
59	23.8	Sopaipilla, without syrup or honey
59	18.4	Tamale, sweet, with fruit
59	24.2	Strudel, apple
59	27.6	Strudel, berry
59	26.6	Strudel, cherry
59	22.2	Baklava
59	25.7	Turnover or dumpling, apple
59	27.0	Turnover or dumpling, berry
59	23.6	Turnover or dumpling, cherry
59	21.9	Turnover or dumpling, lemon
59	24.8	Turnover or dumpling, peach
59	22.1	Turnover, guava
59	15.1	Turnover, pumpkin
59	23.4	Pastry, fruit-filled

GRAIN PRODUCTS

GI	GL	Food Name
59	39.2	Pastry, Oriental, made with bean or lotus seed paste filling (baked)
59	33.1	Pastry, Oriental, made with bean paste and salted egg yolk filling (baked)
59	18.6	Pastry, Italian, with cheese
59	27.0	Pastry, puff
59	17.6	Pastry, puff, custard or cream filled, iced or not iced
59	36.1	Pastry, mainly flour and water, fried
59	29.8	Empanada, Mexican turnover, fruit-filled
59	20.3	Empanada, Mexican turnover, pumpkin
59	26.3	Breakfast pastry
59	26.3	Danish pastry, plain or spice
59	28.2	Danish pastry, with fruit
59	27.0	Danish pastry, with nuts
59	21.9	Danish pastry, with cheese
59	37.9	Danish pastry, with cheese, fat free, cholesterol free
76	35.7	Doughnut, NS as to cake or yeast
76	37.8	Doughnut, cake type
76	43.6	Doughnut, chocolate, cake type
76	36.5	Doughnut, cake type, chocolate covered
76	37.9	Doughnut, cake type, chocolate covered, dipped in peanuts
76	40.1	Doughnut, chocolate, cake type, with chocolate icing
76	34.9	Churros
76	41.0	Doughnut, oriental

GI	GL	Food Name
76	37.8	Cruller
76	45.2	French cruller
76	39.1	Doughnut, chocolate, raised or yeast, with chocolate
76	33.7	Doughnut, raised or yeast
76	34.0	Doughnut, chocolate, raised or yeast
76	38.1	Doughnut, raised or yeast, chocolate covered
76	29.6	Doughnut, jelly
76	22.8	Doughnut, custard-filled
76	29.5	Doughnut, chocolate cream-filled
76	40.5	Doughnut, custard-filled, with icing
76	32.4	Doughnut, wheat
76	42.0	Doughnut, wheat, chocolate covered
70	49.8	Breakfast tart
70	53.8	Breakfast tart, lowfat
57	39.8	Breakfast bar
72	52.5	Breakfast bar, cereal crust with fruit filling, lowfat
72	55.2	Breakfast bar, cereal crust with fruit filling, fat free
54	32.5	Breakfast bar, date, with yogurt coating
39	28.1	Meal replacement bar
61	40.7	Granola bar, oats, sugar, raisins, coconut
61	47.2	Granola bar, oats, fruit and nuts, lowfat
61	47.3	Granola bar, nonfat
61	38.9	Granola bar, peanuts, oats, sugar, wheat germ
62	41.4	Granola bar, chocolate-coated

GI	GL	Food Name
62	34.2	Granola bar, with coconut, chocolate-coated
62	33.5	Granola bar with nuts, chocolate-coated
51	31.2	Granola bar, coated with non-chocolate coating
51	33.4	Granola bar, high fiber, coated with non-chocolate yogurt coating
63	41.0	Granola bar, with rice cereal
56	36.0	PowerBar (fortified high energy bar)
58	30.2	Coffee cake, crumb or quick-bread type
58	43.8	Coffee cake, crumb or quick-bread type, reduced fat, cholesterol free
58	33.9	Coffee cake, crumb or quick-bread type, with fruit
58	22.5	Coffee cake, crumb or quick-bread type, cheese-filled
58	25.7	Coffee cake, crumb or quick-bread type, custard filled

Crackers and Salty Snacks

GI	GL	Food Name
74	45.1	Crackers, NS as to sweet or nonsweet
65	48.2	Cracker, animal
74	56.8	Crackers, graham
74	49.2	Crackers, graham, chocolate covered
74	58.3	Crackers, graham, with raisins
74	59.5	Crackers, graham, lowfat
74	62.2	Crackers, graham, fat free
71	57.6	Crackers, matzo, low sodium
74	52.9	Crackers, saltine, low sodium
74	60.9	Crackers, saltine, fat free, low sodium

GI	GL	Food Name
70	45.4	Crackers, toast thins (rye, wheat, white flour), low sodium
67	46.0	Cracker, 100% whole wheat, low sodium
55	33.6	Cracker, snack, low sodium
55	32.0	Cracker, cheese, low sodium
55	41.5	Cracker, snack, lowfat, low sodium
78	63.6	Puffed rice cake without salt
55	35.0	Cracker, multigrain, salt free
55	45.2	Crispbread, rye, low sodium
55	33.6	Cracker, snack
55	44.9	Cracker, snack, reduced fat
55	45.8	Cracker, snack, fat free
55	32.0	Cracker, cheese
55	39.4	Cracker, cheese, reduced fat
55	44.2	Cracker, high fiber, no added fat
55	46.5	Crispbread, wheat, no added fat
64	47.5	Crispbread, wheat or rye, extra crispy
71	59.4	Crackers, matzo
55	38.3	Crackers, milk
71	50.3	Crackers, oyster
78	63.3	Rice cake, cracker-type
78	58.0	Crackers, rice
78	63.6	Puffed rice cake
64	52.6	Crispbread, rye, no added fat
74	52.5	Crackers, saltine

GRAIN PRODUCTS

GI	GL	Food Name
67	46.7	Crackers, saltine, whole wheat
59	28.4	Crackers, cylindrical, peanut-butter filled
59	33.5	Crackers, sandwich-type
59	34.4	Cracker, sandwich-type, peanut butter filled
70	45.4	Crackers, toast thins (rye, pumpernickel, white flour)
71	50.9	Crackers, water biscuits
67	46.0	Cracker, 100% whole wheat
67	47.5	Cracker, 100% whole wheat, reduced fat
67	45.9	Crackers, whole wheat and bran
67	43.5	Crackers, wheat
67	48.6	Crackers, wheat, reduced fat
63	45.3	Salty snacks, corn or cornmeal base, nuts or nuggets, toasted
63	39.7	Salty snacks, corn or cornmeal base, corn chips, corn-cheese chips
63	34.1	Salty snacks, corn or cornmeal base, corn puffs and twists; corn-cheese puffs and twists
63	41.2	Salty snacks, corn or cornmeal base, tortilla chips
63	36.2	Salty snacks, corn or cornmeal base, corn chips, corn-cheese chips, unsalted
63	46.2	Salty snacks, corn or cornmeal base, tortilla chips, light (baked with less oil)
63	50.4	Salty snacks, corn or cornmeal base, tortilla chips, lowfat, baked without fat
63	50.5	Salty snacks, corn or cornmeal base, tortilla chips, lowfat, baked without fat, unsalted

GI	GL	Food Name
63	41.2	Salty snacks, corn or cornmeal base, with oat bran, tortilla chips
63	45.6	Salty snacks, corn based puffs and twists, cheese puffs and twists, lowfat
63	41.2	Salty snacks, corn or cornmeal base, tortilla chips, unsalted
63	40.1	Salty snack mixture, mostly corn or cornmeal based, with pretzels, without nuts
63	41.1	Salty snacks, wheat-based, high fiber
63	40.5	Salty snacks, wheat- and corn-based chips
63	40.0	Salty snacks, multigrain, chips
72	41.4	Popcorn, popped in oil, unbuttered
72	56.0	Popcorn, air-popped (no butter or no oil added)
72	37.4	Popcorn, popped in oil, buttered
72	38.6	Popcorn, air-popped, buttered
72	37.4	Popcorn, flavored
72	52.8	Popcorn, popped in oil, lowfat, low sodium
72	52.0	Popcorn, popped in oil, lowfat
72	41.8	Popcorn, popped in oil, unsalted
83	66.2	Pretzels
83	66.2	Pretzels, hard
83	57.6	Pretzels, soft
83	65.7	Pretzel, hard, unsalted
83	60.6	Pretzel, oatbran, hard
83	65.2	Pretzel, hard, multigrain

GRAIN PRODUCTS

GI	GL	Food Name
83	49.4	Multigrain mixture, bread sticks, sesame nuggets, pretzels, rye chips
72	53.9	Bagel chip

Pancakes, Waffles, Other Grain Products

GI	GL	Food Name
67	26.3	Pancakes, plain
67	24.9	Pancakes, reduced calorie, high fiber
67	17.9	Pancakes, with fruit
102	24.8	Pancakes, buckwheat
67	21.2	Pancakes, cornmeal
67	19.5	Pancakes, whole wheat
67	22.7	Pancakes, sour dough
67	31.7	Pancakes, rye
76	37.1	Waffle, plain
76	33.7	Waffle, wheat, bran, or multigrain
76	34.0	Waffle, fruit
76	31.4	Waffle, nut and honey
76	29.0	Waffle, cornmeal
76	25.3	Waffle, 100% whole wheat or 100% whole grain
76	31.2	Waffle, oat bran
76	27.4	Waffle, multi-bran
76	38.1	Waffle, plain, fat free
76	36.7	Waffle, plain, lowfat
67	20.6	French toast, plain
67	27.5	French toast sticks, plain

GI	GL	Food Name
67	14.5	Crepe, plain
50	8.4	Flour and water gravy
64	32.9	Cake made with glutinous rice
76	24.5	Funnel cake

Pastas, Cooked Cereals, Rice

GI	GL	Food Name
47	14.4	Macaroni, cooked
47	14.4	Macaroni, cooked, fat not added in cooking
47	14.0	Macaroni, cooked, fat added in cooking
37	9.8	Macaroni, whole wheat, cooked
37	9.8	Macaroni, whole wheat, cooked, fat not added in cooking
37	9.5	Macaroni, whole wheat, cooked, fat added in cooking
47	12.8	Macaroni, cooked, spinach
47	12.8	Macaroni, cooked, spinach, fat not added in cooking
47	12.4	Macaroni, cooked, spinach, fat added in cooking
47	12.5	Macaroni, cooked, vegetable
47	12.5	Macaroni, cooked, vegetable, fat not added in cooking
47	12.1	Macaroni, cooked, vegetable, fat added in cooking
42	10.5	Noodles, cooked, fat not added in cooking
42	10.2	Noodles, cooked, fat added in cooking
37	8.7	Noodles, cooked, whole wheat
37	9.8	Noodles, cooked, whole wheat, fat not added in cooking
42	10.1	Noodles, cooked, spinach
42	10.1	Noodles, cooked, spinach, fat not added in cooking
42	9.9	Noodles, cooked, spinach, fat added in cooking

GRAIN PRODUCTS

GI	GL	Food Name
50	28.8	Noodles, chow mein
33	6.8	Long rice noodles (made from mung beans) cooked
33	6.8	Long rice noodles (made from mung beans), cooked, fat not added in cooking
33	6.6	Long rice noodles (made from mung beans), cooked, fat added in cooking
51	11.8	Chow fun rice noodles, cooked
51	11.8	Chow fun rice noodles, cooked, fat not added in cooking
51	11.5	Chow fun rice noodles, cooked, fat added in cooking
42	12.9	Spaghetti, cooked
42	12.9	Spaghetti, cooked, fat not added in cooking
42	12.5	Spaghetti, cooked, fat added in cooking
42	12.9	Spaghetti, cooked, high protein type (assume no fat added)
25	7.0	Barley, cooked
25	7.0	Barley, cooked, fat not added in cooking
45	8.9	Buckwheat groats, cooked
45	8.9	Buckwheat groats, cooked, fat not added in cooking
45	8.6	Buckwheat groats, cooked, fat added in cooking
69	6.8	Grits, cooked, corn or hominy
69	6.6	Grits, cooked, corn or hominy, fat not added in cooking
69	6.8	Grits, cooked, corn or hominy, regular, fat not added in cooking
69	6.6	Grits, cooked, corn or hominy, regular, fat added in cooking

GI	GL	Food Name
69	6.6	Grits, cooked, corn or hominy, regular
69	6.6	Grits, cooked, corn or hominy, fat added in cooking
69	6.5	Grits, cooked, corn or hominy, with cheese
69	8.7	Grits, cooked, corn or hominy, quick, fat not added in cooking
69	8.2	Grits, cooked, corn or hominy, quick, fat added in cooking
69	8.5	Grits, cooked, corn or hominy, quick
69	10.4	Grits, cooked, corn or hominy, instant, fat not added in cooking
69	9.8	Grits, cooked, corn or hominy, instant, fat added in cooking
69	10.4	Grits, cooked, corn or hominy, instant
69	9.6	Grits, cooked, flavored, corn or hominy, instant, fat not added in cooking
69	9.1	Grits, cooked, flavored, corn or hominy, instant, fat added in cooking
69	9.6	Grits, cooked, flavored, corn or hominy, instant
69	10.0	Grits, cooked, corn or hominy, made with milk
89	17.5	Cornmeal mush, made with water
56	11.9	Cornmeal mush, made with milk
76	18.8	Cornmeal dumpling
76	23.2	Cornmeal sticks, boiled
69	14.1	Cornmeal, lime-treated, cooked (Masa harina)
71	16.7	Millet, cooked, fat not added in cooking
58	6.3	Oatmeal, cooked

GRAIN PRODUCTS

GI	GL	Food Name
58	6.3	Oatmeal, cooked, quick (1 or 3 minutes)
58	6.3	Oatmeal, cooked, regular
58	6.3	Oatmeal, cooked, fat not added in cooking
58	6.3	Oatmeal, cooked, regular, fat not added in cooking
58	6.3	Oatmeal, cooked, quick (1 or 3 minutes), fat not added in cooking
58	10.6	Oatmeal, cooked, instant, fat not added in cooking
58	6.1	Oatmeal, cooked, fat added in cooking
58	6.1	Oatmeal, cooked, regular, fat added in cooking
58	6.1	Oatmeal, cooked, quick (1 or 3 minutes), fat added in cooking
58	10.2	Oatmeal, cooked, instant, fat added in cooking
58	10.6	Oatmeal, cooked, instant
58	7.7	Oatmeal with maple flavor, cooked
58	9.4	Oatmeal with fruit, cooked
48	6.8	Oatmeal, made with milk, fat not added in cooking
48	6.8	Oatmeal, made with milk
53	9.4	Oatmeal, made with evaporated milk and sugar, Puerto Rican style
58	8.1	Oatmeal, multigrain, cooked
58	8.1	Oatmeal, multigrain, cooked, fat not added in cooking
47	12.1	Rice, white, cooked, converted
64	17.9	Rice, white, cooked, regular
64	17.7	Rice, cooked
64	17.9	Rice, white, cooked, regular, fat not added in cooking

GI	GL	Food Name
69	17.2	Rice, white, cooked, instant
69	17.2	Rice, white, cooked, instant, fat not added in cooking
47	12.1	Rice, white, cooked, converted, fat not added in cooking
64	7.3	Rice, cream of, cooked, fat not added in cooking
55	12.5	Rice, brown, cooked, regular, fat not added in cooking
55	12.5	Rice, brown, cooked, regular
64	13.4	Yellow rice, cooked, regular
64	13.4	Yellow rice, cooked, regular, fat not added in cooking
64	13.1	Yellow rice, cooked, regular, fat added in cooking
98	20.7	Rice, white, cooked, glutinous
57	12.1	Rice, wild, 100%, cooked, fat not added in cooking
54	11.3	Rice, white and wild, cooked, fat not added in cooking
54	11.0	Rice, brown and wild, cooked, fat not added in cooking
54	11.1	Rice, white and wild, cooked, fat added in cooking
54	11.1	Rice, white and wild, cooked
54	10.8	Rice, brown and wild, cooked, fat added in cooking
54	10.8	Rice, brown and wild, cooked
64	17.4	Rice, cooked, fat added in cooking
64	23.4	Rice, white, cooked with (fat) oil, Puerto Rican style (Arroz blanco)
64	17.4	Rice, white, cooked, regular, fat added in cooking
69	16.7	Rice, white, cooked, instant, fat added in cooking
47	11.8	Rice, white, cooked, converted, fat added in cooking
55	12.3	Rice, brown, cooked, regular, fat added in cooking

GRAIN PRODUCTS

GI	GL	Food Name
55	12.5	Rice, brown, cooked, instant
64	14.6	Rice, brown, cooked, instant, fat not added in cooking
64	14.3	Rice, brown, cooked, instant, fat added in cooking
66	6.0	Wheat, cream of, cooked, quick
66	6.0	Wheat, cream of, cooked, regular
66	6.0	Wheat, cream of, cooked
66	6.0	Wheat, cream of, cooked, fat not added in cooking
66	6.0	Wheat, cream of, cooked, regular, fat not added in cooking
66	6.0	Wheat, cream of, cooked, quick, fat not added in cooking
74	8.5	Wheat, cream of, cooked, instant, fat not added in cooking
50	5.9	Wheat, cream of, cooked, made with milk
74	8.1	Wheat, cream of, cooked, instant, fat added in cooking
74	8.5	Wheat, cream of, cooked, instant
48	8.9	Bulgur, cooked or canned, fat not added in cooking
48	8.4	Bulgur, cooked or canned, fat added in cooking
48	8.9	Bulgur, cooked or canned
65	15.0	Couscous, plain, cooked, fat not added in cooking
65	15.0	Couscous, plain, cooked
65	14.2	Couscous, plain, cooked, fat added in cooking
48	4.9	Whole wheat cereal, cooked
48	4.9	Whole wheat cereal, cooked, fat not added in cooking
48	4.8	Whole wheat cereal, cooked, fat added in cooking

GI	GL	Food Name
66	5.8	Wheat, cream of, cooked, regular, fat added in cooking
66	5.9	Wheat, cream of, cooked, quick, fat added in cooking
37	5.5	Whole wheat cereal, wheat and barley, cooked, fat not added in cooking
37	5.5	Whole wheat cereal, wheat and barley, cooked
55	4.9	Oat bran cereal, cooked, fat not added in cooking
55	4.8	Oat bran cereal, cooked, fat added in cooking
44	6.0	Oat bran cereal, cooked, made with milk, fat not added in cooking

Other Cereals

GI	GL	Food Name
75	61.9	Cereal
74	59.2	Kashi cereal
74	55.9	Oat cereal
75	61.9	Cereal, ready-to-eat
42	31.2	All-Bran
42	32.3	All-Bran with Extra Fiber
74	62.2	Apple Cinnamon Cheerios
58	46.5	Apple Cinnamon Squares Mini-Wheats, Kellogg's (formerly Apple Cinnamon Squares)
113	98.3	Berry Berry Kix
58	46.4	All-Bran Bran Buds, Kellogg's (formerly Bran Buds)
58	48.7	Bran Chex
74	54.8	Cheerios
58	49.3	Chex cereal
80	69.8	Chocolate flavored frosted puffed corn cereal

GRAIN PRODUCTS

GI	GL	Food Name
77	66.3	Cocoa Krispies
77	67.7	Puffed rice cereal with cocoa (Includes: Cocoa Pebbles)
80	70.4	Cocoa Puffs
77	59.3	Complete Oat Bran Flakes, Kellogg's (formerly Common Sense Oat Bran, plain)
75	64.8	Crunchy Corn Bran, Quaker
83	71.4	Corn Chex
81	70.4	Corn flakes
81	70.6	Corn flakes, Kellogg
81	69.7	Corn Puffs
81	69.3	Total Corn Flakes
77	55.0	Cracklin' Oat Bran
87	74.8	Crispix
82	70.5	Crispy Brown Rice Cereal
82	70.7	Crispy Rice
61	49.4	Crispy Wheats'n Raisins
42	34.0	Fiber One
74	57.8	Fiber 7 Flakes, Health Valley
74	59.2	Bran Flakes (formerly 40% Bran Flakes)
74	58.5	Complete Wheat Bran Flakes, Kellogg's (formerly 40% Bran Flakes)
74	59.5	Bran flakes cereal (Includes: Post Natural Bran Flakes, formerly called 40% Bran Flakes)
69	60.4	Froot Loops
74	63.6	Frosted Cheerios

GI	GL	Food Name
58	46.6	Frosted Mini-Wheats
72	60.3	Shredded wheat cereal, presweetened (Includes: Frosted Wheat Bites)
42	32.0	Fruit & Fibre (fiber)
69	60.4	Fruit Rings
71	58.9	Golden Grahams
71	57.7	Wheat and malt barley cereal, granules (Includes: Grape-Nuts)
80	65.2	Wheat and malt barley cereal, flakes (Includes: Grape-Nuts Flakes)
68	53.4	Healthy Choice Almond Crunch with raisins, Kellogg's
77	63.1	Corn, whole wheat and rolled oats cereal
77	60.1	Corn, whole wheat and rolled oats cereal with almonds
72	62.6	Honey Crunch Corn Flakes, Kellogg's
74	59.2	Honey Nut Cheerios
71	63.2	Smacks, Kellogg's (formerly Honey Smacks)
60	50.2	Just Right
60	49.0	Just Right Fruit and Nut (formerly Just Right with raisins, dates, and nuts)
74	59.2	Kashi, Puffed
81	69.7	Kix
66	51.5	Life (plain and cinnamon)
77	68.9	Malt-O-Meal Coco-Roos
82	70.1	Malt-O-Meal Crispy Rice
74	59.2	Malt-O-Meal Honey and Nut Toasty O's

GRAIN PRODUCTS

GI	GL	Food Name
87	76.4	Malt-O-Meal Puffed Rice
74	56.5	Malt-O-Meal Puffed Wheat
71	63.2	Malt-O-Meal Golden Puffs (formerly Sugar Puffs)
74	54.8	Malt-O-Meal Toasted Oat Cereal
69	60.7	Malt-O-meal Tootie Fruities
107	85.6	Millet, puffed
48	35.8	Mueslix cereal
49	38.1	Muesli with raisins, dates, and almonds
58	48.7	Multi Bran Chex
74	59.9	Multi Grain Cheerios
71	57.7	Nutty Nuggets, Ralston Purina
67	52.7	Oat Bran Flakes, Health Valley
77	58.5	Oatmeal Crisp with Almonds
71	59.5	Oh's, Honey Graham
42	32.8	Bran and malted flour cereal (Includes: 100% Bran)
76	63.1	Product 19
55	41.2	Quaker Oat Bran Cereal
77	60.3	Quaker Oatmeal Squares (formerly Quaker Oat Squares)
61	46.6	Raisin bran
61	46.5	Raisin Bran, Kellogg
61	46.9	Raisin Bran, Post
61	45.8	Raisin Bran, Total
65	51.9	Raisin Mini-Wheats, Kellogg's (formerly Raisin Squares Mini-Wheats; Raisin Squares)

GI	GL	Food Name
89	76.5	Rice Chex
82	70.1	Rice Krispies
82	71.3	Rice Krispies Treats Cereal (Kellogg's)
87	76.4	Rice, puffed
61	48.7	Shredded wheat and bran cereal (Includes: Shredded Wheat'N Bran)
69	49.0	Special K
77	59.6	Oatmeal Honey Nut Heaven, Quaker (formerly Toasted Oatmeal, Honey Nut)
80	72.0	Corn Pops
72	57.6	Strawberry Squares Mini-Wheats, Kellogg's (formerly Strawberry Squares)
55	49.7	Frosted corn flakes
55	49.7	Frosted Flakes, Kellogg
71	64.5	Puffed wheat cereal, presweetened (Includes: Golden Crisp, formerly called Super Golden Crisp)
74	54.9	Toasted oat cereal
74	55.2	Malt-O-Meal Toasty O's
76	57.0	Total
42	27.6	Uncle Sam's Hi Fiber Cereal
70	54.2	Weetabix Whole Wheat Cereal
58	47.0	Wheat Chex
74	56.5	Wheat, puffed, plain
71	63.9	Wheat, puffed, presweetened with sugar
75	60.7	Shredded wheat, plain (Includes: Shredded Wheat,

GRAIN PRODUCTS

GI	GL	Food Name
37	30.0	Wheaties
34	8.3	Burrito with beef and beans
34	6.9	Burrito with beef, beans, and cheese
30	8.0	Burrito with beef and cheese, no beans
33	6.5	Burrito with beef, beans, cheese, and sour cream
34	9.8	Burrito with beans and cheese, meatless
31	5.8	Burrito with eggs, sausage, cheese and vegetables
68	14.0	Taco or tostada with beef, cheese and lettuce
58	7.6	Taco or tostada with beef, cheese, lettuce, tomato and salsa
30	7.7	Soft taco with beef, cheese, and lettuce
55	8.3	Taco or tostada with beans, cheese, meat, lettuce, tomato and salsa
56	5.5	Taco or tostada salad with beef and cheese, corn chips
31	5.7	Fajita with chicken and vegetables
60	18.2	Pizza, cheese
60	17.7	Pizza, cheese, thin crust
60	19.0	Pizza, cheese, thick crust
49	14.4	Pizza, cheese, with vegetables
49	12.4	Pizza, cheese, with vegetables, thin crust
49	16.5	Pizza, cheese, with vegetables, thick crust
60	22.2	Pizza, cheese, with fruit, thick crust
30	9.4	Pizza with meat
30	8.1	Pizza with meat, thin crust

GI	GL	Food Name
36	12.9	Pizza with meat, thick crust
30	8.2	Pizza with meat and vegetables
30	7.0	Pizza with meat and vegetables, thin crust
36	11.4	Pizza with meat and vegetables, thick crust
30	7.4	Pizza with meat and fruit, thin crust
36	11.8	Pizza with meat and fruit, thick crust
30	6.5	Pizza with meat and vegetables, lowfat, thin crust
80	35.2	Pizza, no cheese, thick crust
60	21.7	Italian pie, meatless
50	7.6	Egg roll, meatless
50	7.6	Egg roll, with shrimp
50	7.2	Egg roll, with beef and/or pork
50	7.3	Egg roll, with chicken or turkey
52	15.0	Dumpling, potato- or cheese-filled
68	5.8	Gnocchi, cheese
46	8.8	Lasagna, meatless
39	7.4	Ravioli, no sauce
39	5.6	Ravioli, with tomato sauce
39	6.8	Ravioli, meat-filled, no sauce
39	5.5	Ravioli, meat-filled, with tomato sauce or meat sauce
59	7.9	Ravioli, meat-filled, with tomato sauce or meat sauce, canned
50	10.1	Ravioli, cheese-filled, no sauce
44	6.7	Ravioli, cheese-filled, with tomato sauce

GRAIN PRODUCTS

GI	GL	Food Name
39	5.4	Ravioli, cheese-filled, with meat sauce
40	8.6	Spaghetti with tomato sauce, meatless
40	5.9	Pasta with tomato sauce and cheese, canned
52	9.7	Spaghetti with tomato sauce and meatballs or spaghetti with meat sauce or spaghetti with meat sauce and meatballs
52	6.4	Pasta with tomato sauce and meat or meatballs, canned
52	8.9	Spaghetti with tomato sauce and meatballs, whole wheat noodles or spaghetti with meat sauce, whole wheat noodles or spaghetti with meat sauce and meatballs, whole wheat noodles
40	7.4	Spaghetti with tomato sauce, meatless, made with spinach noodles
52	8.1	Spaghetti with tomato sauce and frankfurters or hot dogs
40	7.5	Spaghetti with clam sauce
40	7.1	Spaghetti with red clam sauce
42	7.8	Spaghetti with white clam sauce
52	10.4	Spaghetti with tomato sauce and chicken or turkey
50	7.6	Tortellini, cheese-filled, meatless, with tomato sauce
50	8.8	Tortellini, cheese-filled, meatless, with vinaigrette dressing
50	7.8	Tortellini, cheese-filled, with cream sauce
51	7.2	Chow fun noodles with meat and vegetables
64	13.7	Macaroni or noodles with cheese
64	7.4	Macaroni or noodles with cheese, canned
64	16.5	Macaroni or noodles with cheese, made from dry mix

GI	GL	Food Name
64	16.0	Macaroni or noodles with cheese, from boxed mix with already prepared cheese sauce
40	9.4	Macaroni or noodles with cheese and tomato
40	6.7	Pasta with tomato sauce, meatless
52	6.8	Pasta with meat sauce
52	6.7	Pasta with cheese and meat sauce
42	10.8	Pasta with carbonara sauce
40	6.5	Pasta with cheese and tomato sauce, meatless
36	6.9	Macaroni or noodles with beans or lentils and tomato sauce
51	9.8	Macaroni, creamed
43	10.5	Macaroni, creamed, with cheese
42	6.9	Macaroni, creamed, with vegetables
42	6.1	Flavored pasta
45	10.3	Macaroni or pasta salad
46	8.8	Pasta or macaroni salad with oil and vinegar-type
65	20.2	Noodle pudding
64	13.8	Rice pilaf
56	10.7	Dirty rice
55	11.1	Flavored rice mixture
54	10.5	Flavored rice, brown and wild
64	11.4	Rice dressing
38	1.8	Soup
42	1.6	Noodle soup

GRAIN PRODUCTS

GI	GL	Food Name
64	2.3	Rice soup
25	1.8	Barley soup
42	1.5	Beef noodle soup
64	3.0	Beef rice soup
42	1.4	Beef noodle soup, home recipe
42	1.3	Chicken noodle soup
42	1.9	Chicken noodle soup, canned, low sodium, ready-to-
42	1.2	Chicken noodle soup, home recipe
35	1.9	Chicken noodle soup, cream of
42	1.5	Chicken noodle soup, canned, reduced sodium, ready-to-serve
42	2.7	Noodle and potato soup, Puerto Rican style
64	1.9	Chicken rice soup
64	3.8	Chicken or turkey rice soup, home recipe
64	2.2	Chicken rice soup, canned, reduced sodium, prepared with water or ready-to-serve
64	8.0	Rice and potato soup, Puerto Rican style
42	1.5	Turkey noodle soup
42	1.4	Turkey noodle soup, home recipe
42	1.3	Instant soup, noodle
42	4.2	Soup, mostly noodles
64	2.3	Instant soup, rice
42	4.0	Instant soup, noodle with egg, shrimp or chicken
40	2.5	Noodle soup with vegetables, Oriental style

GI	GL	Food Name
42	3.0	Noodle soup, with fish ball, shrimp, and dark green leafy vegetable

FRUITS

Citrus Fruits, Juices

GI	GL	Food Name
25	2.0	Grapefruit, raw
25	2.3	Grapefruit, canned or frozen, unsweetened, water pack
25	3.9	Grapefruit, canned or frozen, in light syrup
48	33.4	Lemon pie filling
42	4.9	Orange, raw
42	6.8	Orange, mandarin, canned or frozen, in light syrup
42	4.0	Orange, mandarin, canned or frozen, drained
42	4.9	Tangelo, raw
42	5.6	Tangerine, raw
48	4.4	Grapefruit juice, freshly squeezed
48	4.3	Grapefruit juice
48	4.3	Grapefruit juice, canned, bottled or in a carton
48	4.6	Grapefruit juice, frozen (reconstituted with water)
50	5.5	Orange juice
50	5.2	Orange juice, freshly squeezed
50	4.9	Orange juice, canned, bottled or in a carton
50	4.9	Orange juice, with calcium added, canned, bottled or in a carton
50	5.5	Orange juice, frozen (reconstituted with water)
50	19.1	Orange juice, frozen, not reconstituted

FRUITS

GI	GL	Food Name
50	5.4	Orange juice, frozen, with calcium added (reconstituted with water)
50	6.5	Grape-tangerine-lemon juice
49	5.0	Grapefruit and orange juice
49	4.8	Grapefruit and orange juice, fresh
49	5.0	Grapefruit and orange juice, canned
50	6.9	Orange and banana juice
48	5.9	Pineapple-orange-banana juice
50	6.0	Orange-white grape-peach juice
50	6.1	Apricot-orange juice
47	5.1	Pineapple-grapefruit juice, canned, bottled or in a carton, unsweetened
48	5.5	Pineapple-orange juice
48	5.5	Pineapple-orange juice, canned, bottled or in a carton
48	5.7	Pineapple-orange juice, frozen (reconstituted)
50	6.2	Strawberry-banana-orange juice

Dried Fruits

GI	GL	Food Name
38	25.5	Fruit, dried (assume uncooked)
38	24.8	Fruit mixture, dried (mixture includes three or more of the following: apples, apricots, dates, papaya, peaches, pears, pineapples, prunes, raisins)
29	19.1	Apple, dried, uncooked
29	4.4	Apple, dried, cooked
29	6.7	Apple, dried, cooked, with sugar
29	21.4	Apple chips

GI	GL	Food Name
31	19.4	Apricot, dried, uncooked
31	6.9	Apricot, dried, cooked
31	6.9	Apricot, dried, cooked, unsweetened
31	9.1	Apricot, dried, cooked, with sugar
64	47.4	Currants, dried
103	77.3	Date
61	39.0	Fig, dried, uncooked
61	20.7	Fig, dried, cooked, with sugar
29	18.5	Prune, dried, uncooked
29	8.1	Prune, dried, cooked
29	8.1	Prune, dried, cooked, unsweetened
29	10.1	Prune, dried, cooked, with sugar
64	50.7	Raisins
64	36.7	Raisins, cooked

Other Fruits

GI	GL	Food Name
38	5.2	Apple, raw
38	7.6	Applesauce, stewed apples
38	4.3	Applesauce, stewed apples, unsweetened
38	7.6	Applesauce, stewed apples, with sugar
38	4.3	Applesauce, stewed apples, sweetened with low calorie sweetener
38	6.4	Apple, cooked or canned, with syrup
38	5.6	Apple, baked, unsweetened
38	9.4	Apple, baked, with sugar

FRUITS

GI	GL	Food Name
38	12.2	Apple, pickled
38	9.2	Apple, fried
57	6.3	Apricot, raw
64	13.7	Apricot, cooked or canned
64	4.1	Apricot, cooked or canned, unsweetened, water pack
64	13.7	Apricot, cooked or canned, in heavy syrup
64	10.6	Apricot, cooked or canned, in light syrup
64	13.6	Apricot, cooked or canned, drained solids
50	4.3	Avocado, raw
52	11.9	Banana, raw
52	11.9	Banana, red, ripe (guineo morado)
52	13.4	Banana, ripe, fried
52	11.9	Banana, ripe, boiled
65	5.3	Cantaloupe (muskmelon), raw
48	13.8	Cherry pie filling
22	2.0	Cherries, sour, red, cooked, unsweetened
22	3.5	Cherries, sweet, raw (Queen Anne, Bing)
22	4.7	Cherries, sweet, cooked or canned
22	4.7	Cherries, sweet, cooked or canned, in heavy syrup
22	3.8	Cherries, sweet, cooked or canned, in light syrup
22	4.6	Cherries, sweet, cooked or canned, drained solids
22	3.0	Cherries, sweet, cooked or canned, juice pack
22	2.4	Cherries, frozen
64	8.8	Currants, raw

GI	GL	Food Name
61	11.7	Fig, raw
61	10.9	Figs, cooked or canned, in light syrup
46	8.3	Grapes, raw, NS as to type
46	8.3	Grapes, European type, adherent skin, raw
46	7.9	Grapes, American type, slip skin, raw
53	7.8	Kiwi fruit, raw
65	5.9	Honeydew melon, raw
65	5.9	Honeydew, frozen (balls)
42	4.4	Nectarine, raw
59	5.8	Papaya, raw
59	4.0	Papaya, green, cooked
59	11.5	Papaya, cooked or canned, in sugar or syrup
42	4.0	Peach, raw
58	11.6	Peach, cooked or canned
38	2.3	Peach, cooked or canned, unsweetened, water pack
58	11.6	Peach, cooked or canned, in heavy syrup
52	7.6	Peach, cooked or canned, in light or medium syrup
42	8.3	Peach, cooked or canned, drained solids
38	4.4	Peach, cooked or canned, juice pack
58	13.9	Peach, frozen, NS as to added sweetener
42	4.0	Peach, frozen, unsweetened
58	13.9	Peach, frozen, with sugar
38	5.9	Pear, raw
38	4.0	Pear, Japanese, raw

FRUITS

GI	GL	Food Name
44	8.3	Pear, cooked or canned
44	8.3	Pear, cooked or canned, in heavy syrup
25	3.8	Pear, cooked or canned, in light syrup
38	7.3	Pear, cooked or canned, drained solids
44	5.6	Pear, cooked or canned, juice pack
59	7.5	Pineapple, raw
59	9.3	Pineapple, cooked or canned
59	4.9	Pineapple, cooked or canned, unsweetened, waterpack
59	11.9	Pineapple, cooked or canned, in heavy syrup
59	7.9	Pineapple, cooked or canned, in light syrup
59	9.2	Pineapple, cooked or canned, drained solids
59	9.3	Pineapple, cooked or canned, juice pack
39	4.5	Plum, raw
39	9.1	Plum, cooked or canned, in heavy syrup
39	6.3	Plum, cooked or canned, in light syrup
72	5.4	Watermelon, raw
40	3.2	Berries, raw
40	5.8	Blueberries, raw
40	3.1	Strawberries, raw
55	6.7	Strawberries, raw, with sugar
55	12.9	Strawberries, cooked or canned
55	12.9	Strawberries, cooked or canned, in syrup
55	12.9	Strawberries, frozen, NS as to added sweetener
40	3.7	Strawberries, frozen, unsweetened

GI	GL	Food Name
55	12.9	Strawberries, frozen, with sugar
55	7.8	Fruit cocktail or mix (excluding citrus fruits), raw
55	7.6	Fruit cocktail or mix (including citrus fruits), raw
55	6.6	Fruit cocktail or mix, frozen
55	10.1	Fruit cocktail, cooked or canned
55	4.7	Fruit cocktail, cooked or canned, unsweetened, water pack
55	10.4	Fruit cocktail, cooked or canned, in heavy syrup
55	8.2	Fruit cocktail, cooked or canned, in light syrup
55	10.3	Fruit cocktail, cooked or canned, drained solids
55	6.5	Fruit cocktail, cooked or canned, juice pack
34	9.6	Apple, candied
54	5.9	Fruit, chocolate covered
49	7.5	Fruit salad (excluding citrus fruits) with salad dressing or mayonnaise
48	7.2	Fruit salad (excluding citrus fruits) with cream
46	8.2	Fruit salad (excluding citrus fruits) with cream substitute
41	5.1	Fruit salad (including citrus fruits) with salad dressing or mayonnaise
50	3.8	Guacamole with tomatoes
50	3.8	Guacamole with tomatoes and chili peppers
50	4.3	Guacamole
59	13.7	Fruit juice bar, frozen, orange flavor
59	11.9	Fruit juice bar, frozen, flavor other than orange

FRUITS

GI	GL	Food Name
59	6.5	Fruit juice bar, frozen, sweetened with low calorie sweetener, flavors other than orange
59	11.9	Sorbet, fruit, noncitrus flavor
59	13.7	Sorbet, fruit, citrus flavor
42	10.1	Fruit juice bar with cream, frozen

Non-Citrus Juices and Nectars

GI	GL	Food Name
50	5.6	Fruit juice
40	5.2	Fruit juice blend, 100% juice, with added Vitamin C
40	4.7	Apple cider
40	4.7	Apple juice
43	5.0	Apple-cherry juice
40	4.7	Apple-pear juice
40	4.4	Apple-raspberry juice
40	5.2	Apple-grape juice
40	5.0	Apple-grape-raspberry juice
68	8.3	Cranberry juice, unsweetened
68	9.4	Cranberry-white grape juice mixture, unsweetened
46	6.9	Grape juice
46	5.9	Pineapple juice
43	5.2	Pineapple-apple-guava juice, with added vitamin C
46	6.0	Pineapple juice-non-citrus juice blend, unsweetened, with added vitamin C
29	5.1	Prune juice, unsweetened

VEGETABLES

White Potatoes and Starchy Vegetables

GI	GL	Food Name
66	12.8	White potato
73	15.5	White potato, baked, peel not eaten
73	14.9	White potato, baked, peel eaten
73	15.2	White potato, baked, peel eaten, fat not added
73	14.9	White potato, baked, peel eaten, fat added in cooking
73	25.5	White potato skins, with adhering flesh, baked
66	12.8	White potato, boiled, without peel
66	13.2	White potato, boiled, without peel, fat not added in cooking
66	12.8	White potato, boiled, without peel, fat added in cooking
48	9.3	White potato, boiled, with peel
66	13.2	White potato, boiled, with peel, fat not added in cooking
48	9.3	White potato, boiled, with peel, fat added in cooking
73	14.5	White potato, roasted
73	15.6	White potato, roasted, fat not added in cooking
73	14.5	White potato, roasted, fat added in cooking
54	26.9	White potato, chips
54	36.1	White potato, chips, reduced fat
54	45.2	White potato, chips, fat free
54	27.5	White potato, chips, restructured
54	35.0	White potato, chips, restructured, reduced fat and reduced sodium
54	38.6	White potato, chips, restructured, baked

VEGETABLES

GI	GL	Food Name
54	28.6	White potato, chips, unsalted
54	36.6	White potato, chips, unsalted, reduced fat
54	28.8	White potato, sticks
54	27.5	White potato skins, chips
67	9.9	White potato, cooked, with sauce, NS as to sauce
69	10.6	White potato, cooked, with cheese
69	10.7	White potato, scalloped
69	9.7	White potato, scalloped, with ham
75	26.7	White potato, french fries
75	25.2	White potato, french fries, from fresh, deep fried
75	22.7	White potato, french fries, from frozen, oven baked
75	28.1	White potato, french fries, from frozen, deep fried
75	23.4	White potato, french fries, breaded or battered
75	17.5	White potato, home fries
75	16.8	White potato, home fries, with green or red peppers and onions
75	26.2	White potato, hash brown
75	26.2	White potato, hash brown, from fresh
75	20.9	White potato, hash brown, from frozen
75	20.9	White potato, hash brown, from dry mix
75	23.5	White potato, hash brown, with cheese
79	12.5	White potato, mashed
79	14.3	White potato, from fresh, mashed, made with milk
79	13.9	White potato, from fresh, mashed, made with milk and

GI	GL	Food Name
79	15.2	White potato, from fresh, mashed, made with fat
85	8.9	White potato, from dry, mashed, made with milk and fat
79	13.4	White potato, from fresh, mashed, made with milk, fat and cheese
85	23.9	White potato, from dry, mashed, made with milk, fat and egg
79	15.8	White potato, from fresh, mashed, not made with milk or fat
85	9.3	White potato, from dry, mashed, made with milk, no fat
85	12.1	White potato, from complete dry mix, mashed, made with water
85	10.4	White potato, from dry, mashed
79	10.5	White potato, from fresh, mashed
70	11.7	White potato, stuffed, baked, peel not eaten
69	10.9	White potato, stuffed, baked, peel not eaten, stuffed with sour cream
69	12.8	White potato, stuffed, baked, peel not eaten, stuffed with cheese
67	12.0	White potato, stuffed, baked, peel not eaten, stuffed with chili
69	11.5	White potato, stuffed, baked, peel not eaten, stuffed with broccoli and cheese sauce
69	8.9	White potato, stuffed, baked, peel not eaten, stuffed with chicken, broccoli and cheese sauce
70	11.5	White potato, stuffed, baked, peel eaten, NS as to
70	11.5	White potato, stuffed, baked, peel eaten, stuffed with sour cream

VEGETABLES

GI	GL	Food Name
70	13.2	White potato, stuffed, baked, peel eaten, stuffed with cheese
70	12.1	White potato, stuffed, baked, peel eaten, stuffed with broccoli and cheese sauce
69	11.5	White potato, stuffed, baked, peel eaten, stuffed with meat in cream sauce
69	12.4	White potato, stuffed, baked, peel not eaten, stuffed with bacon and cheese
66	10.5	Potato salad with egg
68	11.4	Potato salad, German style
66	11.7	Potato salad
65	7.7	Stewed potatoes with tomatoes
50	2.9	Potato soup
50	3.4	Potato soup, cream of, prepared with milk
50	2.3	Potato soup, prepared with water
54	4.8	Potato and cheese soup
63	10.2	Macaroni and potato soup
53	4.1	Potato chowder
39	12.1	Plantain, boiled, NS as to green or ripe
39	14.1	Plantain, fried, NS as to green or ripe
39	12.1	Green plantains, boiled
39	13.6	Fried green plantain, Puerto Rican style (Tostones)
38	8.6	Green banana, cooked (in salt water)
30	7.0	Green banana, fried
46	17.2	Cassava (yuca blanca), cooked

GI	GL	Food Name
46	17.6	Cassava (yuca blanca), cooked, fat not added in cooking
56	39.9	Casabe, cassava bread
37	10.1	Yam, Puerto Rican (Name), cooked
32	11.5	Tannier, cooked
32	11.2	Dasheen, boiled
55	18.7	Taro, baked

Dark Green Vegetables

GI	GL	Food Name
32	1.4	Beet greens, raw
32	1.7	Beet greens, cooked
32	1.3	Chard, cooked
32	1.5	Collards, cooked
32	1.5	Collards, cooked, from fresh
32	1.6	Collards, cooked, from fresh, fat not added in cooking
32	2.3	Collards, cooked, from frozen, fat not added in cooking
32	1.6	Collards, cooked, from canned, fat not added in cooking
32	1.5	Collards, cooked, fat added in cooking
32	1.5	Collards, cooked, from fresh, fat added in cooking
32	2.2	Collards, cooked, from frozen, fat added in cooking
32	1.5	Collards, cooked, from canned, fat added in cooking
32	2.9	Dandelion greens, raw
32	2.0	Dandelion greens, cooked, fat not added in cooking
32	2.0	Dandelion greens, cooked, fat added in cooking
32	1.2	Endive, chicory, escarole, or romaine lettuce, raw

VEGETABLES

GI	GL	Food Name
32	1.4	Escarole, cooked, fat not added in cooking
32	1.5	Escarole, cooked, fat added in cooking
32	1.5	Greens, cooked
32	1.6	Greens, cooked, from fresh, fat not added in cooking
32	1.6	Greens, cooked, from canned, fat not added in cooking
32	1.5	Greens, cooked, fat added in cooking
32	1.5	Greens, cooked, from fresh, fat added in cooking
32	1.7	Kale, cooked
32	1.8	Kale, cooked, from canned
32	1.8	Kale, cooked, from fresh, fat not added in cooking
32	1.8	Kale, cooked, from fresh, fat added in cooking
32	0.7	Mustard greens, cooked, from fresh
32	1.0	Mustard greens, cooked, from frozen
32	0.7	Mustard greens, cooked, fat not added in cooking
32	0.7	Mustard greens, cooked, from fresh, fat not added in cooking
32	1.0	Mustard greens, cooked, from frozen, fat not added in cooking
32	0.7	Mustard greens, cooked, from canned, fat not added in cooking
32	0.7	Mustard greens, cooked, fat added in cooking
32	0.7	Mustard greens, cooked, from fresh, fat added in cooking
32	1.0	Mustard greens, cooked, from frozen, fat added in cooking

GI	GL	Food Name
32	0.7	Mustard greens, cooked, from canned, fat added in cooking
32	1.0	Poke greens, cooked
32	1.0	Poke greens, cooked, fat added in cooking
32	1.4	Radicchio, raw
32	1.2	Spinach, raw
32	1.2	Spinach, cooked
32	1.2	Spinach, cooked, from fresh
32	1.6	Spinach, cooked, from frozen
32	1.1	Spinach, cooked, from canned
32	1.2	Spinach, cooked, fat not added in cooking
32	1.2	Spinach, cooked, from fresh, fat not added in cooking
32	1.6	Spinach, cooked, from frozen, fat not added in cooking
32	1.1	Spinach, cooked, from canned, fat not added in cooking
32	1.2	Spinach, cooked, fat added in cooking
32	1.2	Spinach, cooked, from fresh, fat added in cooking
32	1.6	Spinach, cooked, from frozen, fat added in cooking
32	1.1	Spinach, cooked, from canned, fat added in cooking
28	1.7	Spinach, creamed
29	1.7	Spinach, cooked, from frozen, with cheese sauce
32	2.6	Taro leaves, cooked, fat not added in cooking
32	1.4	Turnip greens, cooked
32	1.4	Turnip greens, cooked, from fresh
32	1.4	Turnip greens, cooked, from canned

VEGETABLES

GI	GL	Food Name
32	1.4	Turnip greens, cooked, fat not added in cooking
32	1.4	Turnip greens, cooked, from fresh, fat not added in cooking
32	1.6	Turnip greens, cooked, from frozen, fat not added in cooking
32	1.4	Turnip greens, cooked, from canned, fat not added in cooking
32	1.4	Turnip greens, cooked, fat added in cooking
32	1.4	Turnip greens, cooked, from fresh, fat added in cooking
32	1.6	Turnip greens, cooked, from frozen, fat added in cooking
32	1.4	Turnip greens, cooked, from canned, fat added in cooking
32	0.9	Turnip greens with roots, cooked, from frozen, fat not added in cooking
32	1.5	Turnip greens with roots, cooked, from fresh, fat added in cooking
32	0.4	Watercress, raw
32	1.5	Sweetpotato leaves, squash leaves, pumpkin leaves, chrysanthemum leaves, bean leaves, or swamp cabbage, cooked, fat not added in cooking
32	2.1	Broccoli, raw
32	2.2	Broccoli, cooked
32	2.2	Broccoli, cooked, from fresh
32	1.7	Broccoli, cooked, from frozen
32	2.3	Broccoli, cooked, fat not added in cooking
32	2.3	Broccoli, cooked, from fresh, fat not added in cooking
32	1.7	Broccoli, cooked, from frozen, fat not added in cooking

GI	GL	Food Name
32	2.2	Broccoli, cooked, fat added in cooking
32	2.2	Broccoli, cooked, from fresh, fat added in cooking
32	1.7	Broccoli, cooked, from frozen, fat added in cooking
29	2.0	Broccoli, cooked, with cheese sauce
29	2.0	Broccoli, cooked, from fresh, with cheese sauce
29	1.7	Broccoli, cooked, from frozen, with cheese sauce
28	2.0	Broccoli, cooked, with cream sauce
28	2.3	Broccoli, cooked, from fresh, with cream sauce
28	2.0	Broccoli, cooked, from frozen, with cream sauce
27	2.0	Broccoli soup
27	1.7	Broccoli cheese soup, prepared with milk
38	0.3	Dark-green leafy vegetable soup with meat, Oriental
38	0.1	Dark-green leafy vegetable soup, meatless, Oriental

Deep Yellow Vegetables

GI	GL	Food Name
16	1.5	Carrots, raw
47	3.8	Carrots, cooked
47	3.8	Carrots, cooked, from fresh
47	3.5	Carrots, cooked, from frozen
47	2.6	Carrots, cooked, from canned
47	3.8	Carrots, cooked, fat not added in cooking
47	3.8	Carrots, cooked, from fresh, fat not added in cooking
47	3.6	Carrots, cooked, from frozen, fat not added in cooking
47	2.6	Carrots, cooked, from canned, fat not added in cooking
47	3.8	Carrots, cooked, fat added in cooking
47	3.8	Carrots, cooked, from fresh, fat added in cooking

VEGETABLES

GI	GL	Food Name
47	3.5	Carrots, cooked, from frozen, fat added in cooking
47	2.6	Carrots, cooked, from canned, fat added in cooking
37	3.2	Carrots, cooked, from fresh, creamed
59	9.2	Carrots, cooked, glazed
59	9.2	Carrots, cooked, from fresh, glazed
47	2.5	Carrots, canned, low sodium, fat not added in cooking
37	3.6	Peas and carrots, creamed
37	3.6	Peas and carrots, from frozen, creamed
48	4.7	Peas and carrots, cooked
48	5.9	Peas and carrots, cooked, from fresh
48	4.7	Peas and carrots, cooked, from frozen
48	4.7	Peas and carrots, cooked, from canned
48	4.8	Peas and carrots, cooked, fat not added in cooking
48	6.0	Peas and carrots, cooked, from fresh, fat not added in cooking
48	4.8	Peas and carrots, cooked, from frozen, fat not added in cooking
48	4.8	Peas and carrots, cooked, from canned, fat not added in cooking
48	4.7	Peas and carrots, cooked, fat added in cooking
48	4.7	Peas and carrots, cooked, from frozen, fat added in cooking
48	4.7	Peas and carrots, cooked, from canned, fat added in cooking
48	4.0	Peas and carrots, canned, low sodium, fat not added in cooking

GI	GL	Food Name
75	3.7	Pumpkin, cooked, fat not added in cooking
75	3.7	Pumpkin, cooked, from fresh, fat not added in cooking
75	6.0	Pumpkin, cooked, from canned, fat not added in cooking
75	3.6	Pumpkin, cooked, from fresh, fat added in cooking
75	6.0	Calabaza (Spanish pumpkin), cooked
75	6.5	Squash, winter type, mashed, NS as to fat or sugar added in cooking
75	6.6	Squash, winter type, mashed, no fat or sugar added in cooking
75	6.5	Squash, winter type, mashed, fat added in cooking, no sugar added in cooking
71	10.0	Squash, winter type, mashed, fat and sugar added in cooking
71	10.0	Squash, winter type, baked, NS as to fat or sugar added in cooking
75	6.6	Squash, winter type, baked, no fat or sugar added in cooking
75	6.5	Squash, winter type, baked, fat added in cooking, no sugar added in cooking
71	10.0	Squash, winter type, baked, fat and sugar added in cooking
71	10.2	Squash, winter type, baked, no fat added in cooking, sugar added in cooking
72	8.8	Squash, winter, souffle
61	12.2	Sweetpotato
61	15.5	Sweetpotato, baked, peel eaten
61	15.9	Sweetpotato, baked, peel eaten, fat not added in

VEGETABLES

GI	GL	Food Name
61	12.1	Sweetpotato, baked, peel not eaten
61	12.5	Sweetpotato, baked, peel not eaten, fat not added in cooking
61	12.1	Sweetpotato, baked, peel not eaten, fat added
61	10.5	Sweetpotato, boiled, without peel
61	10.7	Sweetpotato, boiled, without peel, fat not added in cooking
61	10.5	Sweetpotato, boiled, without peel, fat added in cooking
61	10.7	Sweetpotato, boiled, with peel, fat not added in cooking
61	10.5	Sweetpotato, boiled, with peel, fat added in cooking
63	18.1	Sweetpotato, candied
53	13.3	Sweetpotato with fruit
61	12.8	Sweetpotato, canned, NS as to syrup
61	12.9	Sweetpotato, canned without syrup
61	12.8	Sweetpotato, canned in syrup
61	12.5	Sweetpotato, canned in syrup, fat added in cooking
61	9.2	Sweetpotato, casserole or mashed
61	13.1	Sweetpotato, fried
37	0.9	Carrot soup, cream of, prepared with milk

Tomatoes and Tomato Mixtures

GI	GL	Food Name
38	1.5	Tomatoes, raw
38	1.9	Tomatoes, green, raw
38	1.5	Tomatoes, cooked, from fresh
38	1.5	Tomatoes, cooked, from canned

GI	GL	Food Name
38	1.9	Tomatoes, broiled
38	1.9	Tomatoes, from fresh, broiled
38	4.2	Tomatoes, red, fried
38	4.0	Tomatoes, scalloped
38	2.4	Tomatoes, stewed
38	3.7	Tomatoes, from fresh, stewed
38	2.4	Tomatoes, from canned, stewed
38	1.7	Tomatoes, canned, low sodium
38	5.0	Tomatoes, green, cooked
38	5.0	Tomatoes, green, cooked, from fresh
32	2.7	Tomato, green, pickled
38	21.2	Tomatoes, red, dried
38	1.6	Tomato juice
38	1.7	Tomato and vegetable juice, mostly tomato
38	1.7	Tomato and vegetable juice, mostly tomato, low sodium
38	9.5	Tomato catsup
38	10.6	Tomato catsup, low sodium
38	7.5	Tomato chili sauce (catsup-type)
38	2.4	Salsa
38	1.5	Salsa, red, uncooked
38	2.4	Salsa, red, cooked, not homemade
38	1.7	Salsa, red, cooked, homemade
38	2.2	Green tomato-chile sauce, cooked (Salsa verde)
38	4.3	Tomato sauce

VEGETABLES

GI	GL	Food Name
38	6.0	Tomato sauce, low sodium
38	7.2	Tomato paste
38	3.4	Tomato puree
38	4.3	Spaghetti sauce, meatless
38	4.0	Spaghetti sauce with meat, canned, no extra meat added
38	6.0	Spaghetti sauce, meatless, low sodium
38	3.3	Spaghetti sauce, meatless, fat free
32	11.2	Tomato relish
38	7.9	Cocktail sauce
50	5.0	Tomato and corn, cooked, fat not added in cooking
35	1.4	Tomato and okra, cooked
35	1.5	Tomato and okra, cooked, fat not added in cooking
35	1.4	Tomato and okra, cooked, fat added in cooking
35	1.9	Tomato and onion, cooked
35	1.9	Tomato and onion, cooked, fat not added in cooking
35	1.9	Tomato and onion, cooked, fat added in cooking
48	4.9	Tomato with corn and okra, cooked, fat added in cooking
38	2.8	Tomato soup
36	3.3	Tomato soup, cream of, prepared with milk
38	2.6	Tomato soup, prepared with water
38	5.1	Tomato soup, canned, undiluted
38	2.8	Tomato soup, instant type, prepared with water
38	2.8	Tomato soup, canned, low sodium, ready-to-serve
38	3.3	Tomato beef soup, prepared with water

GI	GL	Food Name
40	3.5	Tomato beef noodle soup, prepared with water
40	4.5	Tomato noodle soup, prepared with water
51	4.5	Tomato rice soup, prepared with water
38	1.5	Tomato vegetable soup, prepared with water
40	2.0	Tomato vegetable soup with noodles, prepared with water

Other Vegetables

GI	GL	Food Name
32	1.5	Sprouts
32	1.2	Alfalfa sprouts, raw
32	5.6	Artichoke, Jerusalem, raw
32	1.2	Asparagus, raw
32	1.9	Bean sprouts, raw (soybean or mung)
32	2.3	Beans, string, green, raw
64	6.1	Beets, raw
32	2.9	Brussels sprouts, raw
32	1.8	Cabbage, green, raw
32	0.7	Cabbage, Chinese, raw
32	2.4	Cabbage, red, raw
7	0.2	Cactus, raw
32	1.7	Cauliflower, raw
32	1.0	Celery, raw
32	1.4	Chives, raw
32	1.2	Cilantro, raw
54	10.2	Corn, raw

VEGETABLES

GI	GL	Food Name
32	0.7	Cucumber, raw
32	10.6	Garlic, raw
32	2.8	Jicama, raw
32	4.5	Leek, raw
32	1.0	Lettuce, raw
32	0.7	Lettuce, Boston, raw
32	1.2	Lettuce, arugula, raw
32	1.0	Mixed salad greens, raw
32	1.0	Mushrooms, raw
32	2.3	Onions, young green, raw
32	3.2	Onions, mature, raw
32	2.0	Parsley, raw
48	6.9	Peas, green, raw
32	2.9	Pepper, hot chili, raw
32	1.5	Pepper, poblano, raw
32	2.1	Pepper, Serrano, raw
32	1.5	Pepper, raw
32	1.5	Pepper, sweet, green, raw
32	1.9	Pepper, sweet, red, raw
32	1.7	Pepper, banana, raw
32	1.1	Radish, raw
32	2.7	Seaweed, raw
32	2.4	Snowpeas (pea pod), raw
32	1.1	Squash, summer, yellow, raw

GI	GL	Food Name
32	1.1	Squash, summer, green, raw
72	4.6	Turnip, raw
32	1.3	Celery juice
44	3.4	Cabbage salad or coleslaw, with dressing
32	1.7	Cabbage, Chinese, salad, with dressing
32	0.8	Cucumber salad with creamy dressing
32	2.1	Cucumber salad made with cucumber, oil, and vinegar
32	1.2	Lettuce, salad with assorted vegetables including tomatoes and/or carrots, no dressing
32	1.0	Lettuce, salad with assorted vegetables excluding tomatoes and carrots, no dressing
32	1.7	Lettuce, salad with avocado, tomato, and/or carrots, with or without other vegetables, no dressing
32	1.2	Lettuce, salad with cheese, tomato and/or carrots, with or without other vegetables, no dressing
32	1.2	Lettuce, salad with egg, tomato, and/or carrots, with or without other vegetables, no dressing
32	1.0	Lettuce salad with egg, cheese, tomato, and/or carrots, with or without other vegetables, no dressing
32	0.8	Lettuce, wilted, with bacon dressing
32	2.0	Seven-layer salad (lettuce salad made with a combination of onion, celery, green pepper, peas, mayonnaise, cheese, eggs, and/or bacon)
32	1.0	Greek Salad
43	5.4	Vegetables, cooked
43	5.5	Vegetables, cooked, fat not added in cooking

VEGETABLES

GI	GL	Food Name
43	5.4	Vegetables, cooked, fat added in cooking
32	12.2	Algae, dried
32	3.5	Artichoke, globe (French), cooked
32	3.5	Artichoke, globe (French), cooked, from fresh
32	2.9	Artichoke, globe (French), cooked, from frozen
32	3.5	Artichoke, globe (French), cooked, from canned
32	3.6	Artichoke, globe (French), cooked, fat not added in cooking
32	3.6	Artichoke, globe (French), cooked, from fresh, fat not added in cooking
32	3.5	Artichoke, globe (French), cooked, from fresh, fat added in cooking
32	3.3	Artichoke salad in oil
32	1.3	Asparagus, cooked
32	1.3	Asparagus, cooked, from fresh
32	0.8	Asparagus, cooked, from canned
32	1.3	Asparagus, cooked, fat not added in cooking
32	1.3	Asparagus, cooked, from fresh, fat not added in cooking
32	0.6	Asparagus, cooked, from frozen, fat not added in cooking
32	0.8	Asparagus, cooked, from canned, fat not added in
32	1.3	Asparagus, cooked, fat added in cooking
32	1.3	Asparagus, cooked, from fresh, fat added in cooking
32	0.6	Asparagus, cooked, from frozen, fat added in cooking
32	0.8	Asparagus, cooked, from canned, fat added in cooking
32	1.7	Bamboo shoots, cooked, fat not added in cooking

GI	GL	Food Name
32	2.2	Bamboo shoots, cooked, fat added in cooking
32	7.3	Beans, lima, immature, cooked
32	6.0	Beans, lima, immature, cooked, from frozen
32	7.3	Beans, lima, immature, cooked, from canned
32	7.5	Beans, lima, immature, cooked, fat not added in cooking
32	7.5	Beans, lima, immature, cooked, from fresh, fat not added in cooking
32	6.2	Beans, lima, immature, cooked, from frozen, fat not added in cooking
32	7.5	Beans, lima, immature, cooked, from canned, fat not added in cooking
32	7.3	Beans, lima, immature, cooked, fat added in cooking
32	7.3	Beans, lima, immature, cooked, from fresh, fat added in cooking
32	6.0	Beans, lima, immature, cooked, from frozen, fat added in cooking
32	7.3	Beans, lima, immature, cooked, from canned, fat added in cooking
32	4.2	Beans, lima, immature, canned, low sodium
32	2.4	Beans, string, cooked, fat added in cooking
32	2.4	Beans, string, cooked, from fresh, fat added in cooking
32	2.0	Beans, string, cooked, from frozen, fat added in cooking
32	1.4	Beans, string, cooked, from canned, fat added in cooking
32	2.5	Beans, string, cooked, fat not added in cooking
32	2.5	Beans, string, cooked, from fresh, fat not added in

VEGETABLES

GI	GL	Food Name
32	2.0	Beans, string, cooked, from frozen, fat not added in cooking
32	1.4	Beans, string, cooked, from canned, fat not added in cooking
32	2.4	Beans, string, cooked
32	2.4	Beans, string, cooked, from fresh
32	2.0	Beans, string, cooked, from frozen
32	1.4	Beans, string, cooked, from canned
32	2.4	Beans, string, green, cooked
32	2.4	Beans, string, green, cooked, from fresh
32	2.0	Beans, string, green, cooked, from frozen
32	1.4	Beans, string, green, cooked, from canned
32	2.5	Beans, string, green, cooked, fat not added in cooking
32	2.5	Beans, string, green, cooked, from fresh, fat not added in cooking
32	2.0	Beans, string, green, cooked, from frozen, fat not added in cooking
32	1.4	Beans, string, green, cooked, from canned, fat not added in cooking
32	2.4	Beans, string, green, cooked, fat added in cooking
32	2.4	Beans, string, green, cooked, from fresh, fat added in cooking
32	2.0	Beans, string, green, cooked, from frozen, fat added in cooking
32	1.4	Beans, string, green, cooked, from canned, fat added in cooking

GI	GL	Food Name
32	1.4	Beans, string, green, canned, low sodium
32	1.4	Beans, string, green, canned, low sodium, fat not added in cooking
32	1.4	Beans, string, green, canned, low sodium, fat added in cooking
32	1.4	Beans, string, yellow, cooked, from canned
32	2.5	Beans, string, yellow, cooked, fat not added in cooking
32	2.5	Beans, string, yellow, cooked, from fresh, fat not added in cooking
32	2.0	Beans, string, yellow, cooked, from frozen, fat not added in cooking
32	1.4	Beans, string, yellow, cooked, from canned, fat not added in cooking
32	2.4	Beans, string, yellow, cooked, from fresh, fat added in cooking
32	1.4	Beans, string, yellow, cooked, from canned, fat added in cooking
32	1.6	Bean sprouts, cooked
32	1.6	Bean sprouts, cooked, from fresh
32	1.7	Bean sprouts, cooked, from fresh, fat not added in cooking
32	0.7	Bean sprouts, cooked, from canned, fat not added in cooking
32	1.6	Bean sprouts, cooked, fat added in cooking
32	1.6	Bean sprouts, cooked, from fresh, fat added in cooking
32	0.7	Bean sprouts, cooked, from canned, fat added in cooking
64	6.2	Beets, cooked

VEGETABLES

GI	GL	Food Name
64	6.2	Beets, cooked, from fresh
64	4.5	Beets, cooked, from canned
64	6.3	Beets, cooked, fat not added in cooking
64	6.3	Beets, cooked, from fresh, fat not added in cooking
64	4.6	Beets, cooked, from canned, fat not added in cooking
64	6.2	Beets, cooked, fat added in cooking
64	4.5	Beets, cooked, from canned, fat added in cooking
32	1.4	Bitter melon, cooked, fat not added in cooking
68	20.4	Breadfruit, cooked, fat not added in cooking
32	2.0	Broccoflower, cooked, fat not added in cooking
32	2.0	Broccoflower, cooked, fat added in cooking
32	2.2	Brussels sprouts, cooked, from fresh
32	2.3	Brussels sprouts, cooked, fat not added in cooking
32	2.3	Brussels sprouts, cooked, from fresh, fat not added in cooking
32	2.6	Brussels sprouts, cooked, from frozen, fat not added in cooking
32	2.6	Brussels sprouts, cooked, from frozen, fat added in cooking
32	0.7	Cabbage, Chinese, cooked
32	0.8	Cabbage, Chinese, cooked, fat not added in cooking
32	0.7	Cabbage, Chinese, cooked, fat added in cooking
32	1.4	Cabbage, green, cooked
32	1.4	Cabbage, green, cooked, fat not added in cooking
32	1.4	Cabbage, green, cooked, fat added in cooking

GI	GL	Food Name
32	2.2	Cabbage, red, cooked
32	2.2	Cabbage, red, cooked, fat not added in cooking
32	2.2	Cabbage, red, cooked, fat added in cooking
7	0.2	Cactus, cooked
7	0.2	Cactus, cooked, fat not added in cooking
7	0.2	Cactus, cooked, fat added in cooking
32	1.2	Cauliflower, cooked
32	1.3	Cauliflower, cooked, from fresh
32	1.2	Cauliflower, cooked, from frozen
32	1.3	Cauliflower, cooked, fat not added in cooking
32	1.3	Cauliflower, cooked, from fresh, fat not added in cooking
32	1.2	Cauliflower, cooked, from frozen, fat not added in
32	1.2	Cauliflower, cooked, fat added in cooking
32	1.3	Cauliflower, cooked, from fresh, fat added in cooking
32	1.2	Cauliflower, cooked, from frozen, fat added in cooking
32	1.3	Celery, cooked
32	1.3	Celery, cooked, fat not added in cooking
32	1.3	Celery, cooked, fat added in cooking
32	1.4	Christophine, cooked, fat not added in cooking
54	13.0	Corn, cooked
54	13.0	Corn, cooked, from fresh
47	8.8	Corn, cooked, from frozen
46	8.3	Corn, cooked, from canned
54	13.4	Corn, cooked, fat not added in cooking

VEGETABLES

GI	GL	Food Name
54	13.4	Corn, cooked, from fresh, fat not added in cooking
47	9.0	Corn, cooked, from frozen, fat not added in cooking
46	8.6	Corn, cooked, from canned, fat not added in cooking
54	13.0	Corn, cooked, fat added in cooking
54	13.0	Corn, cooked, from fresh, fat added in cooking
47	8.8	Corn, cooked, from frozen, fat added in cooking
46	8.3	Corn, cooked, from canned, fat added in cooking
54	9.7	Corn, cream style
46	8.3	Corn, from canned, cream style
54	13.0	Corn, yellow, cooked
54	13.0	Corn, yellow, cooked, from fresh
47	8.8	Corn, yellow, cooked, from frozen
46	8.3	Corn, yellow, cooked, from canned
54	13.4	Corn, yellow, cooked, fat not added in cooking
54	13.4	Corn, yellow, cooked, from fresh, fat not added in cooking
47	9.0	Corn, yellow, cooked, from frozen, fat not added in cooking
46	8.6	Corn, yellow, cooked, from canned, fat not added in cooking
54	13.0	Corn, yellow, cooked, fat added in cooking
54	13.0	Corn, yellow, cooked, from fresh, fat added in cooking
47	8.8	Corn, yellow, cooked, from frozen, fat added in cooking
46	8.3	Corn, yellow, cooked, from canned, fat added in cooking
54	9.7	Corn, yellow, cream style

GI	GL	Food Name
46	8.3	Corn, yellow, from canned, cream style
54	13.0	Corn, yellow and white, cooked
54	13.0	Corn, yellow and white, cooked, from fresh
47	8.9	Corn, yellow and white, cooked, from frozen
54	13.4	Corn, yellow and white, cooked, fat not added in cooking
54	13.4	Corn, yellow and white, cooked, from fresh, fat not added in cooking
47	9.1	Corn, yellow and white, cooked, from frozen, fat not added in cooking
46	8.6	Corn, yellow and white, cooked, from canned, fat not added in cooking
54	13.0	Corn, yellow and white, cooked, from fresh, fat added in cooking
46	8.2	Corn, yellow, from canned, cream style, fat added in cooking
54	13.0	Corn, white, cooked
54	13.0	Corn, white, cooked, from fresh
46	8.3	Corn, white, cooked, from canned
54	13.4	Corn, white, cooked, fat not added in cooking
54	13.4	Corn, white, cooked, from fresh, fat not added in cooking
47	9.1	Corn, white, cooked, from frozen, fat not added in
46	8.6	Corn, white, cooked, from canned, fat not added in cooking
54	13.0	Corn, white, cooked, from fresh, fat added in cooking
47	8.9	Corn, white, cooked, from frozen, fat added in cooking
46	8.3	Corn, white, cooked, from canned, fat added in cooking

VEGETABLES

GI	GL	Food Name
46	8.3	Corn, white, from canned, cream style
46	11.6	Corn, yellow, canned, low sodium, fat not added in cooking
46	11.3	Corn, yellow, canned, low sodium, fat added in cooking
32	1.1	Cucumber, cooked
32	1.4	Cucumber, cooked, fat not added in cooking
32	1.1	Cucumber, cooked, fat added in cooking
32	2.7	Eggplant, cooked
32	2.8	Eggplant, cooked, fat not added in cooking
32	2.7	Eggplant, cooked, fat added in cooking
32	10.6	Garlic, cooked
40	5.4	Hominy, cooked
40	5.7	Hominy, cooked, fat not added in cooking
40	5.4	Hominy, cooked, fat added in cooking
32	5.1	Lotus root, cooked, fat not added in cooking
32	1.7	Mushrooms, cooked
32	1.7	Mushrooms, cooked, from fresh
32	1.7	Mushrooms, cooked, from frozen
32	1.6	Mushrooms, cooked, from canned
32	1.7	Mushrooms, cooked, fat not added in cooking
32	1.7	Mushrooms, cooked, from fresh, fat not added in cooking
32	1.6	Mushrooms, cooked, from canned, fat not added in cooking
32	1.7	Mushrooms, cooked, fat added in cooking

GI	GL	Food Name
32	1.7	Mushrooms, cooked, from fresh, fat added in cooking
32	1.7	Mushrooms, cooked, from frozen, fat added in cooking
32	1.6	Mushrooms, cooked, from canned, fat added in cooking
32	4.6	Mushroom, Oriental, cooked, from dried
32	1.6	Okra, cooked
32	1.4	Okra, cooked, from fresh
32	1.8	Okra, cooked, from frozen
32	1.7	Okra, cooked, fat not added in cooking
32	1.4	Okra, cooked, from fresh, fat not added in cooking
32	1.8	Okra, cooked, from frozen, fat not added in cooking
32	1.4	Okra, cooked, from canned, fat not added in cooking
32	1.6	Okra, cooked, fat added in cooking
32	1.4	Okra, cooked, from fresh, fat added in cooking
32	1.8	Okra, cooked, from frozen, fat added in cooking
32	1.4	Okra, cooked, from canned, fat added in cooking
32	0.9	Lettuce, cooked, fat not added in cooking
32	3.2	Onions, mature, cooked
32	3.2	Onions, mature, cooked, from fresh
32	2.1	Onions, mature, cooked, from frozen
32	3.2	Onions, mature, cooked, fat not added in cooking
32	3.2	Onions, mature, cooked, from fresh, fat not added in cooking
32	2.1	Onions, mature, cooked, from frozen, fat not added in cooking

VEGETABLES

GI	GL	Food Name
32	3.2	Onions, mature, cooked or sauteed, fat added in cooking
32	3.2	Onions, mature, cooked or sauteed, from fresh, fat added in cooking
32	2.1	Onions, mature, cooked or sauteed, from frozen, fat added in cooking
32	3.2	Onions, pearl, cooked
32	3.2	Onions, pearl, cooked, from fresh
32	3.2	Onions, pearl, cooked, from canned
32	2.4	Onion, young green, cooked
32	2.4	Onion, young green, cooked, from fresh
32	2.5	Onions, young green, cooked, fat not added in cooking
32	2.5	Onions, young green, cooked, from fresh, fat not added in cooking
32	2.4	Onion, young green, cooked, fat added in cooking
32	2.4	Onion, young green, cooked, from fresh, fat added in cooking
32	8.2	Palm hearts, cooked (assume fat not added in cooking)
32	2.0	Parsley, cooked (assume fat not added in cooking)
97	16.4	Parsnips, cooked, fat not added in cooking
97	16.0	Parsnips, cooked, fat added in cooking
42	8.3	Peas, cowpeas, field peas, or blackeye peas (not dried), cooked
42	8.3	Peas, cowpeas, field peas, or blackeye peas (not dried), cooked, from fresh
42	8.3	Peas, cowpeas, field peas, or blackeye peas (not dried), cooked, from canned

GI	GL	Food Name
42	8.5	Peas, cowpeas, field peas, or blackeye peas (not dried), cooked, fat not added in cooking
42	8.5	Peas, cowpeas, field peas, or blackeye peas (not dried), cooked, from fresh, fat not added in cooking
42	9.9	Peas, cowpeas, field peas, or blackeye peas (not dried), cooked, from frozen, fat not added in cooking
42	8.5	Peas, cowpeas, field peas, or blackeye peas (not dried), cooked, from canned, fat not added in cooking
42	8.3	Peas, cowpeas, field peas, or blackeye peas (not dried), cooked, fat added in cooking
42	8.3	Peas, cowpeas, field peas, or blackeye peas (not dried), cooked, from fresh, fat added in cooking
42	9.7	Peas, cowpeas, field peas, or blackeye peas (not dried), cooked, from frozen, fat added in cooking
42	8.3	Peas, cowpeas, field peas, or blackeye peas (not dried), cooked, from canned, fat added in cooking
48	7.3	Peas, green, cooked
48	7.3	Peas, green, cooked, from fresh
48	6.6	Peas, green, cooked, from frozen
48	5.9	Peas, green, cooked, from canned
48	7.5	Peas, green, cooked, fat not added in cooking
48	7.5	Peas, green, cooked, from fresh, fat not added in cooking
48	6.8	Peas, green, cooked, from frozen, fat not added in
48	6.0	Peas, green, cooked, from canned, fat not added in cooking
48	7.3	Peas, green, cooked, fat added in cooking
48	7.3	Peas, green, cooked, from fresh, fat added in cooking

VEGETABLES

GI	GL	Food Name
48	6.6	Peas, green, cooked, from frozen, fat added in cooking
48	5.9	Peas, green, cooked, from canned, fat added in cooking
48	4.7	Peas, green, canned, low sodium, fat not added in
22	4.3	Pigeon peas, cooked, fat not added in cooking
32	2.1	Peppers, green, cooked
32	2.1	Peppers, green, cooked, fat not added in cooking
32	2.1	Peppers, green, cooked, fat added in cooking
32	2.1	Peppers, red, cooked, fat not added in cooking
32	3.2	Peppers, hot, cooked
32	3.2	Peppers, hot, cooked, from fresh
32	3.2	Peppers, hot, cooked, from canned
32	3.2	Peppers, hot, cooked, fat not added in cooking
32	3.2	Peppers, hot, cooked, from fresh, fat not added in
32	3.2	Peppers, hot, cooked, from frozen, fat not added in cooking
32	3.2	Peppers, hot, cooked, from canned, fat not added in cooking
32	3.1	Peppers, hot, cooked, fat added in cooking
32	3.1	Peppers, hot, cooked, from fresh, fat added in cooking
32	3.1	Peppers, hot, cooked, from canned, fat added in cooking
32	2.0	Pimiento
32	1.4	Radish, Japanese (daikon), cooked, fat not added in cooking
72	6.3	Rutabaga, cooked, fat not added in cooking
72	6.1	Rutabaga, cooked, fat added in cooking

GI	GL	Food Name
32	1.4	Sauerkraut, cooked
32	1.4	Sauerkraut, cooked, fat not added in cooking
32	1.4	Sauerkraut, cooked, fat added in cooking
32	1.4	Sauerkraut, canned, low sodium
32	2.2	Snowpea (pea pod), cooked
32	2.8	Snowpea (pea pod), cooked, from frozen
32	2.2	Snowpea (pea pod), cooked, fat not added in cooking
32	2.2	Snowpea (pea pod), cooked, from fresh, fat not added in cooking
32	2.9	Snowpea (pea pod), cooked, from frozen, fat not added in cooking
32	2.2	Snowpea (pea pod), cooked, fat added in cooking
32	2.2	Snowpea (pea pod), cooked, from fresh, fat added in cooking
32	2.8	Snowpea (pea pod), cooked, from frozen, fat added in cooking
32	16.8	Seaweed, dried
32	2.5	Seaweed, prepared with soy sauce
32	1.4	Squash, summer, cooked
32	1.4	Squash, summer, cooked, from fresh
32	0.9	Squash, summer, cooked, from canned
32	1.4	Squash, summer, cooked, fat not added in cooking
32	1.4	Squash, summer, cooked, from fresh, fat not added in cooking
32	1.4	Squash, summer, cooked, from frozen, fat not added in cooking

VEGETABLES

GI	GL	Food Name
32	0.9	Squash, summer, cooked, from canned, fat not added in cooking
32	1.4	Squash, summer, cooked, fat added in cooking
32	1.4	Squash, summer, cooked, from fresh, fat added in
32	1.4	Squash, summer, cooked, from frozen, fat added in cooking
32	0.9	Squash, summer, cooked, from canned, fat added in cooking
32	2.0	Squash, spaghetti, cooked
32	2.1	Squash, spaghetti, cooked, fat not added in cooking
72	3.6	Turnip, cooked, from fresh
72	3.6	Turnip, cooked, fat not added in cooking
72	3.6	Turnip, cooked, from fresh, fat not added in cooking
72	3.6	Turnip, cooked, fat added in cooking
72	3.6	Turnip, cooked, from fresh, fat added in cooking
32	3.9	Water chestnut
32	1.0	Winter melon, cooked
43	8.3	Beans, lima and corn (succotash), cooked
35	2.7	Beans, green string, with tomatoes, cooked, fat not added in cooking
32	2.3	Beans, green string, with onions, cooked, fat not added in cooking
63	8.6	Beans, green, and potatoes, cooked, fat not added in cooking
38	2.4	Beans, green, with pinto beans, cooked, fat not added in cooking

GI	GL	Food Name
32	3.2	Bean salad, yellow and/or green string beans
32	2.8	Beans, green string, with onions
32	2.8	Beans, green string, with onions, fat added in cooking
63	8.3	Beans, green, and potatoes, cooked, fat added in cooking
54	12.4	Corn with peppers, red or green, cooked, fat not added in cooking
35	2.8	Eggplant in tomato sauce, cooked, fat not added in cooking
32	2.7	Green peppers and onions, cooked, fat added in cooking
43	5.4	Mixed vegetables (corn, lima beans, peas, green beans, and carrots), cooked
41	5.2	Mixed vegetables (corn, lima beans, peas, green beans, and carrots), cooked, from frozen
41	3.7	Mixed vegetables (corn, lima beans, peas, green beans, and carrots), cooked, from canned
43	5.5	Mixed vegetables (corn, lima beans, peas, green beans, and carrots), cooked, fat not added in cooking
43	5.5	Mixed vegetables (corn, lima beans, peas, green beans, and carrots), cooked, from frozen, fat not added in cooking
43	3.9	Mixed vegetables (corn, lima beans, peas, green beans, and carrots), cooked, from canned, fat not added in cooking
43	5.4	Mixed vegetables (corn, lima beans, peas, green beans, and carrots), cooked, fat added in cooking
41	5.2	Mixed vegetables (corn, lima beans, peas, green beans, and carrots), cooked, from frozen, fat added in cooking

VEGETABLES

GI	GL	Food Name
41	3.7	Mixed vegetables (corn, lima beans, peas, green beans, and carrots), cooked, from canned, fat added in cooking
43	3.1	Mixed vegetables (corn, lima beans, peas, green beans, and carrots), canned, low sodium, fat not added in cooking
51	10.1	Peas and corn, cooked
51	10.4	Peas and corn, cooked, fat not added in cooking
40	3.4	Peas and onions, cooked
40	3.4	Peas and onions, cooked, fat not added in cooking
40	3.4	Peas and onions, cooked, fat added in cooking
47	5.8	Peas with mushrooms, cooked, fat not added in cooking
63	11.2	Peas and potatoes, cooked, fat not added in cooking
32	2.1	Squash, summer, and onions, cooked, fat not added in cooking
35	1.4	Zucchini with tomato sauce, cooked, fat not added in cooking
32	2.0	Squash, summer, and onions, cooked, fat added in cooking
62	6.4	Vegetables, stew type (including potatoes, carrots, onions, celery) cooked, fat added in cooking
62	6.7	Vegetables, stew type (including potatoes, carrots, onions, celery) cooked, fat not added in cooking
32	2.4	Vegetable combinations, Oriental style, (broccoli, green pepper, water chestnut, etc) cooked
32	2.4	Vegetable combinations, Oriental style, (broccoli, green pepper, water chestnuts, etc), cooked, fat not added in cooking

GI	GL	Food Name
32	2.4	Vegetable combinations, Oriental style, (broccoli, green pepper, water chestnuts, etc), cooked, fat added in cooking
49	4.1	Vegetable combinations (broccoli, carrots, corn, cauliflower, etc.), cooked
49	4.2	Vegetable combinations (broccoli, carrots, corn, cauliflower, etc.), cooked, fat not added in cooking
49	4.1	Vegetable combinations (broccoli, carrots, corn, cauliflower, etc.), cooked, fat added in cooking
32	1.9	Vegetable combination (green beans, broccoli, onions, mushrooms), cooked
32	1.9	Vegetable combination (green beans, broccoli, onions, mushrooms), cooked, fat not added in cooking
29	1.5	Asparagus, from fresh, creamed or with cheese sauce
28	1.0	Asparagus, from canned, creamed or with cheese sauce
31	4.6	Beans, lima, immature, from frozen, creamed or with cheese sauce
31	4.7	Beans, lima, immature, cooked, from canned, with mushroom sauce
30	2.2	Beans, string, green, creamed or with cheese sauce
30	1.6	Beans, string, green, from canned, creamed or with cheese sauce
29	1.8	Beans, string, green, cooked, with mushroom sauce
29	1.8	Beans, string, green, cooked, from frozen, with mushroom sauce
29	1.6	Beans, string, green, cooked, from canned, with mushroom sauce
66	14.5	Beets with Harvard sauce

VEGETABLES

GI	GL	Food Name
29	2.3	Brussels sprouts, creamed
29	2.5	Brussels sprouts, from frozen, creamed
28	1.5	Cauliflower, creamed
28	1.5	Cauliflower, from fresh, creamed
28	1.3	Cauliflower, from frozen, creamed
35	2.0	Chiles rellenos, cheese-filled (stuffed chili peppers)
46	7.9	Corn, cooked, with cream sauce, made with milk
46	7.9	Corn, cooked, from fresh, with cream sauce, made with milk
46	6.6	Corn, cooked, from frozen, with cream sauce, made with milk
30	2.9	Onions, creamed
30	2.9	Onions, from fresh, creamed
39	5.0	Peas, from fresh, creamed
39	4.7	Peas, from frozen, creamed
39	4.3	Peas, from canned, creamed
29	1.8	Squash, summer, from fresh, creamed
40	2.7	Turnips, from fresh, creamed
48	4.7	Vegetable combination (including carrots, broccoli, and/or dark-green leafy), cooked, with soy-based sauce
49	6.5	Vegetable combination (excluding carrots, broccoli, and dark-green leafy), cooked, with soy-based sauce
38	3.9	Vegetable combinations (including carrots, broccoli, and/or dark-green leafy), cooked, with cheese sauce
43	5.7	Vegetable combinations (excluding carrots, broccoli, and dark-green leafy), cooked, with cheese sauce

GI	GL	Food Name
30	2.4	Vegetable combination (including carrots, broccoli, and/or dark-green leafy), cooked, with cream sauce
66	9.7	Beets, pickled
54	10.3	Corn relish
32	3.2	Cauliflower, pickled
32	1.8	Cabbage, fresh, pickled, Japanese style
32	11.9	Cabbage, red, pickled
32	1.3	Cabbage, Kim Chee style
32	1.3	Cucumber pickles, dill
32	11.2	Cucumber pickles, relish
32	0.7	Cucumber pickles, sour
32	10.2	Cucumber pickles, sweet
32	6.0	Cucumber pickles, fresh
32	3.1	Eggplant, pickled
32	8.5	Mustard pickles
32	0.7	Cucumber pickles, dill, reduced salt
32	0.9	Mushrooms, pickled
32	2.0	Okra, pickled
50	2.7	Olives
50	1.9	Olives, green
50	3.0	Olives, black
50	2.0	Olives, green, stuffed
32	2.9	Peppers, pickled
32	3.7	Pepper, hot, pickled

VEGETABLES

GI	GL	Food Name
32	1.3	Pickles, NS as to vegetable
32	1.7	Radishes, pickled, Hawaiian style
32	1.2	Recaito (Puerto Rican little coriander)
32	2.8	Vegetable relish
32	1.8	Vegetables, pickled
27	1.5	Asparagus soup, cream of
27	1.8	Asparagus soup, cream of, prepared with milk
27	1.7	Cauliflower soup, cream of, prepared with milk
27	1.3	Celery soup, cream of
27	1.6	Celery soup, cream of, prepared with milk
27	1.0	Celery soup, cream of, prepared with water
41	3.9	Corn soup, cream of, prepared with milk
41	2.7	Corn soup, cream of, prepared with water
27	1.7	Cucumber soup, cream of, prepared with milk
27	2.0	Leek soup, cream of, prepared with milk
27	1.5	Mushroom soup, cream of, prepared with milk
27	0.9	Mushroom soup, cream of, prepared with water
27	1.2	Mushroom soup, cream of, low sodium, prepared with water
27	1.2	Mushroom soup, cream of
27	1.4	Mushroom soup, cream of, canned, reduced sodium
27	1.7	Mushroom soup, cream of, canned, reduced sodium, prepared with milk
27	1.1	Mushroom soup, cream of, canned, reduced sodium, prepared with water

GI	GL	Food Name
27	2.2	Mushroom soup, cream of, canned, reduced sodium, undiluted
66	7.0	Pea soup
47	5.9	Pea soup, prepared with milk
66	7.0	Pea soup, prepared with water
66	7.0	Pea soup, canned, low sodium, prepared with water
33	2.9	Vegetable soup, cream of, prepared with milk
27	1.6	Zucchini soup, cream of, prepared with milk
38	2.1	Vegetable soup, prepared with water or ready-to-serve
38	4.1	Vegetable soup, canned, undiluted
38	2.3	Vegetable soup, canned, low sodium, prepared with water or ready-to-serve
38	1.2	Vegetable soup, made from dry mix
33	2.8	Vegetable soup, cream of, made from dry mix, low sodium, prepared with water
38	1.9	Vegetable soup, home recipe
40	2.5	Vegetable noodle soup, home recipe
39	3.5	Minestrone soup, canned, reduced sodium, ready-to-serve
39	3.6	Minestrone soup, home recipe
39	1.8	Vegetable bean soup, prepared with water or ready-to-serve
38	1.6	Vegetable beef soup, prepared with water
40	2.0	Vegetable noodle soup, prepared with water
38	1.4	Vegetable chicken or turkey soup, prepared with water or ready-to-serve

VEGETABLES

GI	GL	Food Name
51	4.2	Vegetable rice soup, prepared with water
51	3.0	Vegetable beef soup with rice, prepared with water or ready-to-serve
38	3.3	Vegetable chicken soup, canned, low sodium, prepared with water
51	1.7	Vegetable chicken rice soup, prepared with water or ready-to-serve
40	1.3	Vegetable chicken noodle soup, prepared with water or ready-to-serve
38	2.6	Vegetable soup with chicken broth, Mexican style (Sopa Ranchera)
40	3.4	Vegetable noodle soup, canned, reduced sodium, prepared with water or ready-to-serve
38	2.7	Vegetable beef soup, home recipe
38	3.1	Vegetable beef soup, canned, undiluted
40	3.6	Vegetable beef soup with noodles or pasta, home recipe
51	4.3	Vegetable beef soup with rice, home recipe
38	1.9	Vegetarian vegetable soup, prepared with water
38	3.0	Vegetable soup, chunky style
40	3.5	Vegetable soup, with pasta, chunky style
38	2.7	Vegetable beef soup, chunky style

OILS and SALAD DRESSINGS

50	0.0	Butter
50	0.0	Butter, stick, salted
50	0.0	Butter, whipped, tub, salted
50	0.0	Butter, whipped, stick, salted

GI	GL	Food Name
50	0.0	Butter, stick, unsalted
50	0.0	Butter, whipped, tub, unsalted
0	0.0	Light butter, stick, salted
0	0.0	Light butter, stick, unsalted
0	0.0	Light butter, whipped, tub, salted
0	0.0	Margarine
50	1.0	Margarine, stick, salted
50	0.3	Margarine, tub, salted
0	0.0	Margarine, liquid, salted
50	0.3	Margarine, whipped, tub, salted
50	0.5	Margarine, stick, unsalted
0	0.0	Margarine-like spread, stick, salted
50	0.3	Margarine, tub, unsalted
50	0.3	Margarine, whipped, tub, unsalted
0	0.0	Margarine-like spread, tub, salted
0	0.0	Margarine-like spread, liquid, salted
0	0.0	Margarine-like spread, stick, unsalted
0	0.0	Margarine-like spread, tub, unsalted
0	0.0	Margarine-like spread, whipped, tub, salted
50	8.4	Margarine-like spread, tub, sweetened
50	0.2	Margarine-like spread, reduced calorie, about 40% fat, tub, salted
0	0.0	Margarine-like spread, reduced calorie, about 40% fat, stick, salted

OILS and SALAD DRESSINGS

GI	GL	Food Name
0	0.0	Margarine-like spread, reduced calorie, about 20% fat, tub, salted
0	0.0	Margarine-like spread, reduced calorie, about 20% fat, tub, unsalted
50	2.2	Margarine-like spread, fat free, tub, salted
50	1.3	Margarine-like spread, fat free, liquid, salted
50	0.0	Vegetable oil-butter spread, stick, salted
50	0.5	Vegetable oil-butter spread, tub, salted
0	0.0	Vegetable oil-butter spread, reduced calorie, stick,
50	0.5	Vegetable oil-butter spread, reduced calorie, tub, salted
50	0.5	Butter-margarine blend, stick, salted
50	0.3	Butter-margarine blend, tub, salted
50	0.3	Butter-margarine blend, stick, unsalted
50	0.3	Butter-vegetable oil blend
0	0.0	Animal fat or drippings
0	0.0	Lard
0	0.0	Shortening, NS as to vegetable or animal
0	0.0	Shortening, vegetable
0	0.0	Shortening, animal
0	0.0	Ghee, clarified butter
50	11.2	Sandwich spread
55	27.2	Honey butter
0	0.0	Vegetable oil
0	0.0	Almond oil

GI	GL	Food Name
0	0.0	Coconut oil
0	0.0	Corn oil
0	0.0	Corn and canola oil
0	0.0	Cottonseed oil
0	0.0	Flaxseed oil
0	0.0	Olive oil
0	0.0	Peanut oil
0	0.0	Rapeseed oil
0	0.0	Canola and soybean oil
0	0.0	Canola, soybean and sunflower oil
0	0.0	Safflower oil
0	0.0	Sesame oil
0	0.0	Soybean oil
0	0.0	Soybean and sunflower oil
0	0.0	Sunflower oil
0	0.0	Walnut oil
0	0.0	Wheat germ oil
50	4.5	Salad dressing
50	3.7	Blue or roquefort cheese dressing
50	0.3	Bacon dressing (hot)
50	1.6	Caesar dressing
50	11.9	Coleslaw dressing
50	1.1	Feta Cheese Dressing
50	7.8	French dressing

OILS and SALAD DRESSINGS

GI	GL	Food Name
50	22.3	Honey mustard dressing
50	5.2	Italian dressing, made with vinegar and oil
50	2.0	Mayonnaise, regular
50	4.1	Mayonnaise, made with yogurt
50	1.9	Mayonnaise, made with tofu
50	8.0	Mayonnaise, imitation
50	15.5	Russian dressing
50	12.0	Mayonnaise-type salad dressing
50	0.2	Mayonnaise-type salad dressing, cholesterol-free
50	7.5	Boiled, cooked-type dressing
50	3.7	Green Goddess dressing
50	2.4	Creamy dressing, made with sour cream and/or buttermilk and oil
50	2.8	Cream cheese dressing
50	10.8	Milk, vinegar, and sugar dressing
50	10.4	Poppy seed dressing
50	1.8	Peppercorn Dressing
50	10.5	Celery seed dressing
50	4.3	Sesame dressing
50	1.9	Sweet and sour dressing
50	7.3	Thousand Island dressing
50	3.6	Yogurt dressing
50	7.3	Salad dressing, low-calorie
50	1.5	Blue or roquefort cheese dressing, low-calorie

GI	GL	Food Name
50	6.6	Blue or roquefort cheese dressing, reduced calorie
50	12.8	Blue or roquefort cheese dressing, reduced calorie, fat-free, cholesterol-free
50	20.0	Coleslaw dressing, reduced calorie
50	14.6	French dressing, low-calorie
50	16.1	French dressing, reduced calorie, fat-free, cholesterol-
50	13.5	French dressing, reduced calorie
50	9.3	Caesar dressing, low-calorie
50	7.8	Mayonnaise-type salad dressing, fat-free
50	8.0	Mayonnaise, low-calorie or diet
50	8.0	Mayonnaise, low-calorie or diet, low sodium
50	3.4	Mayonnaise, reduced calorie or diet, cholesterol-free
50	12.0	Mayonnaise-type salad dressing, low-calorie or diet
50	12.0	Mayonnaise-type salad dressing, low-calorie or diet, cholesterol-free
50	2.3	Italian dressing, low calorie
50	3.4	Italian dressing, reduced calorie
50	4.4	Italian dressing, reduced calorie, fat-free
50	13.8	Russian dressing, low-calorie
50	11.1	Thousand Island dressing, low-calorie
50	14.6	Thousand Island dressing, reduced calorie, fat-free, cholesterol-free
50	6.1	Vinegar, sugar, and water dressing
50	3.6	Korean dressing or marinade

GI	GL	Food Name
50	3.4	Creamy dressing made with sour cream and/or buttermilk and oil, low calorie
50	10.0	Creamy dressing, made with sour cream and/or buttermilk and oil, reduced calorie, fat-free, cholesterol-free
50	8.0	Creamy dressing, made with sour cream and/or buttermilk and oil, reduced calorie, cholesterol-free
50	2.5	Salad dressing, low calorie, oil-free

SUGARS, SWEETS and BEVERAGES

Sugars and Sweets

68	68.0	Sugar
68	68.0	Sugar, white, granulated or lump
68	67.7	Sugar, white, confectioner's, powdered
68	66.2	Sugar, brown
68	67.1	Sugar, cinnamon
68	66.2	Sugar, raw
19	19.0	Fructose sweetener, sugar substitute, dry powder
50	44.6	Sugar substitute, low-calorie, powdered
50	44.6	Sugar replacement, saccharin-based, dry powder
50	44.6	Sugar substitute, saccharin-based, dry powder and
50	1.0	Sugar substitute, saccharin-based, liquid
50	44.5	Sugar substitute, aspartame-based, dry powder
19	14.6	Corn syrup, light or dark
51	36.6	Fruit syrup

GI	GL	Food Name
19	12.4	Chocolate syrup, thin type
68	22.1	Sugar (white) and water syrup
19	13.2	Maple and corn and/or cane pancake syrup blends (formerly Corn and maple syrup (2% maple))
19	8.4	Syrup, pancake, reduced calorie
55	45.3	Honey
68	46.0	Sugar, brown, liquid
19	13.8	Topping, butterscotch or caramel
19	12.0	Topping, chocolate, thick, fudge type
51	35.7	Jelly, all flavors
51	34.0	Jam, preserves, all flavors
51	21.8	Fruit butter, all flavors
48	31.8	Marmalade, all flavors
55	29.5	Jelly, dietetic, all flavors, sweetened with artificial sweetener
55	25.4	Jelly, reduced sugar, all flavors
55	29.5	Jams, preserves, marmalades, dietetic, all flavors, sweetened with artificial sweetener
51	23.0	Jams, preserves, marmalades, sweetened with fruit juice concentrates, all flavors
55	20.0	Jams, preserves, marmalades, low sugar (all flavors)
68	9.6	Gelatin dessert
60	9.7	Gelatin dessert with fruit
59	19.2	Ice, fruit
68	13.1	Ice pop

SUGARS, SWEETS and BEVERAGES

GI	GL	Food Name
33	20.0	M&M's Almond Chocolate Candies
44	28.9	TWIX Cookie Bars
44	24.6	TWIX Chocolate Fudge Cookie Bars
44	23.2	TWIX Peanut Butter Cookie Bars
43	25.5	Milk chocolate candy, plain
43	27.3	Milk chocolate candy, with cereal
43	22.4	Chocolate, milk, with nuts, not almond or peanuts
43	25.7	Milk chocolate candy, with fruit and nuts
43	22.9	Milk chocolate candy, with almonds
43	23.4	Chocolate, milk, with peanuts
43	27.1	Chocolate, semi-sweet morsel
43	25.6	Chocolate, sweet or dark
44	26.1	Chocolate, white
44	23.5	Chocolate, white, with almonds
44	27.8	Chocolate, white, with cereal
43	25.2	Coconut candy, chocolate covered
43	34.5	Fondant, chocolate covered
99	84.9	Fruit leather
55	35.5	SNICKERS Bar
78	73.0	Licorice
32	29.6	Nougat, plain
65	46.6	Nougat, with caramel, chocolate covered
43	30.8	MILKY WAY Bar
65	40.8	MARS Bar

GI	GL	Food Name
65	54.0	Nougat, chocolate covered
33	20.0	M&M's Peanut Chocolate Candies
33	20.1	M&M's Peanut Butter Chocolate Candies
23	10.9	Peanut bar
23	11.7	Planters Peanut Bar
43	23.8	Reese's Peanut Butter Cup
78	77.1	Gumdrops
70	68.6	Hard candy
70	63.4	Skittles
43	30.6	M&M's Plain Chocolate Candies

Nonalcoholic Beverages

GI	GL	Food Name
50	0.0	Coffee, made from ground, regular
50	0.0	Coffee, made from ground, equal parts regular and decaffeinated
50	0.0	Coffee, espresso
50	0.0	Coffee, espresso, decaffeinated
50	0.0	Coffee, Mexican, regular, unsweetened (no milk; not cafe con leche)
50	0.0	Coffee, Mexican, decaffeinated, unsweetened (no milk; not cafe con leche)
50	0.0	Coffee, made from ground, regular, flavored
68	4.7	Coffee, Cuban
68	2.1	Coffee, latte
50	0.2	Coffee, made from powdered instant, regular

SUGARS, SWEETS and BEVERAGES

GI	GL	Food Name
50	0.3	Coffee, made from powdered instant, 50% less caffeine
50	0.1	Coffee, made from liquid concentrate
50	0.2	Coffee, acid neutralized, from powdered instant
50	0.1	Coffee, decaffeinated, NS as to ground or instant
50	0.0	Coffee, decaffeinated, made from ground
50	0.2	Coffee, decaffeinated, made from powdered instant
48	2.4	Coffee, made from powdered instant mix, with whitener and sugar, instant
68	2.7	Coffee, made from powdered instant mix, presweetened, no whitener
48	2.1	Coffee and cocoa (mocha), made from powdered instant mix, with whitener, presweetened
27	0.6	Coffee and cocoa (mocha), made from powdered instant mix, with whitener and low calorie sweetener
27	1.3	Coffee, made from powdered instant mix, with whitener and low calorie sweetener
27	1.4	Coffee and cocoa (mocha), made from powdered instant mix, with whitener and low calorie sweetener, decaffeinated
57	2.9	Coffee, presweetened with sugar, pre-lightened
32	0.5	Coffee, pre-lightened, no sugar
66	2.7	Coffee, presweetened with sugar
50	0.2	Coffee and chicory, NS as to ground or instant
50	0.2	Coffee, decaffeinated, and chicory, made from powdered instant
50	0.0	Coffee and chicory, made from ground

GI	GL	Food Name
50	0.2	Coffee, decaffeinated, with cereal
68	1.6	Cappuccino
50	0.7	Postum
50	0.5	Cereal beverage
50	0.5	Cereal beverage with beet roots, from powdered instant
50	5.7	Rice beverage
50	0.2	Tea, unsweetened
67	3.5	Tea, presweetened with sugar
50	0.4	Tea, presweetened with low calorie sweetener
50	0.2	Tea, decaffeinated, unsweetened
67	3.6	Tea, presweetened
67	3.6	Tea, decaffeinated, presweetened with sugar
50	0.3	Tea, decaffeinated, presweetened with low calorie sweetener
67	3.6	Tea, decaffeinated, presweetened
50	0.2	Tea, leaf, unsweetened
67	3.6	Tea, leaf, presweetened with sugar
50	0.3	Tea, leaf, presweetened with low calorie sweetener
67	3.6	Tea, leaf, presweetened
50	0.2	Tea, leaf, decaffeinated, unsweetened
67	3.6	Tea, leaf, decaffeinated, presweetened with sugar
50	0.3	Tea, leaf, decaffeinated, presweetened with low calorie sweetener
67	3.6	Tea, leaf, decaffeinated, presweetened

SUGARS, SWEETS and BEVERAGES

GI	GL	Food Name
50	0.2	Tea, made from frozen concentrate, unsweetened
68	5.9	Tea, made from powdered instant, presweetened
50	0.2	Tea, made from powdered instant, unsweetened
68	1.7	Tea, made from powdered instant, presweetened with sugar
68	1.7	Tea, made from powdered instant, decaffeinated, presweetened with sugar
50	0.2	Tea, made from powdered instant, presweetened with low calorie sweetener
50	0.3	Tea, made from powdered instant, decaffeinated, presweetened with low calorie sweetener
50	0.1	Tea, made from powdered instant, decaffeinated, unsweetened
68	1.7	Tea, made from powdered instant, decaffeinated, presweetened
50	0.1	Tea, herbal
50	4.4	Corn beverage
50	0.1	Tea, chamomile
58	5.7	Soft drink
50	0.1	Soft drink, sugar-free
0	0.0	Carbonated water, unsweetened
0	0.0	Carbonated water, sugar-free
58	5.5	Soft drink, cola-type
50	0.1	Soft drink, cola-type, sugar-free
58	6.1	Soft drink, cola-type, with higher caffeine
58	6.1	Soft drink, cola-type, decaffeinated

GI	GL	Food Name
50	0.1	Soft drink, cola-type, decaffeinated, sugar-free
50	0.1	Soft drink, pepper-type, sugar-free
50	0.1	Soft drink, pepper-type, decaffeinated, sugar-free
0	0.0	Cream soda, sugar-free
63	6.4	Soft drink, fruit-flavored, caffeine free
0	0.0	Soft drink, fruit-flavored, sugar free, caffeine free
63	6.6	Soft drink, fruit flavored, caffeine containing
0	0.0	Soft drink, fruit flavored, caffeine containing, sugar-free
0	0.0	Ginger ale, sugar-free
0	0.0	Root beer, sugar-free
50	0.1	Chocolate-flavored soda, sugar-free
58	5.5	Cola with fruit or vanilla flavor
50	0.1	Cola with fruit or vanilla flavor, sugar-free
63	4.4	Carbonated citrus juice drink
59	7.0	Fruit drink
68	7.1	Lemonade
50	2.4	Fruit drink, low calorie
50	0.3	Lemonade, low calorie
59	7.9	Cranberry juice drink with vitamin C added
48	7.6	Cranberry-apple juice drink with vitamin C added
68	8.0	Orange breakfast drink, made from frozen concentrate
68	7.3	Orange breakfast drink
68	6.1	Fruit-flavored drink, made from sweetened powdered mix (fortified with vitamin C)

SUGARS, SWEETS and BEVERAGES

GI	GL	Food Name
50	0.3	Lemonade-flavored drink, made from powdered mix, low calorie
50	0.2	Apple cider-flavored drink, made from powdered mix, low calorie, with vitamin C added
68	8.6	Fruit-flavored drink, made from powdered mix, mainly sugar, with high vitamin C added
68	6.6	Fruit-flavored drink, made from unsweetened powdered mix (fortified with vitamin C), with sugar added in preparation
50	2.8	Apple-white grape juice drink, low calorie, with vitamin C added
50	2.3	Cranberry juice drink, low calorie, with vitamin C added
50	2.4	Cranberry-apple juice drink, low calorie, with vitamin C added
50	1.6	Grapefruit juice drink, low calorie, with vitamin C added
50	2.4	Fruit-flavored drinks, punches, ades, low calorie, with vitamin C added
50	2.4	Juice drink, low calorie
50	1.4	Orange-cranberry juice drink, low calorie, with vitamin C added
50	1.5	Fruit-flavored thirst quencher beverage, low calorie
78	4.9	Fruit-flavored thirst quencher beverage
50	0.2	Fruit-flavored drink, non-carbonated, made from low calorie powdered mix
50	0.6	Wine, light, nonalcoholic
36	2.9	Nonalcoholic malt beverage

Alcoholic Beverages

GI	GL	Food Name
36	1.3	Beer
36	0.6	Beer, lite
50	22.1	Cordial or liqueur
50	0.0	Mixed Drinks (for recipe modifications)
50	10.5	Liqueur with cream
50	1.4	Wine, table, dry
50	2.5	Wine, rice
50	6.8	Wine, dessert, sweet
50	0.6	Wine, light
50	3.3	Wine cooler
50	5.0	Sangria
0	0.0	Brandy
50	0.1	Whiskey
0	0.0	Gin
0	0.0	Rum
0	0.0	Vodka
0	0.0	Water as an ingredient
0	0.0	Water, tap
0	0.0	Water, bottled, unsweetened